Praise for

One-Hundred and Twenty-Six Days

Anyone who has lost a child will relate to Holly Richard's story. It is part memoir, part poetry, part documentary of the Titanic of all cancers—glioblastoma, a primary brain tumor that brought her beautiful young son to his knees and eventually took his life. Holly spares no punches as she documents her family's painful journey in painstaking detail complete with the voices of other families who have gone through the same tragedy. I applaud her courage for sharing her experience which is designed to be cathartic for others in this situation who feel like they are all alone. Richard wants families to know that there is help and support out there for you even in your darkest hour.
—Amanda Lamb, author and journalist

Amanda Lamb, News Reporter
WRAL-TV

Intense love; intense grief. Holly provides a mirror into the depths of a mother's soul who has experienced the gut-wrenching loss of a child to brain cancer. As she mourns the physical absence of her beloved son, Holly walks the reader through her deepest valleys as she struggles to make sense of how to move forward with meaning and purpose in her journey of healing.

Brenda Wilcox RN, MSN, AOCNS, AGCNS-BC Oncology Clinical Nurse Specialist/Transitional Care Navigator Cancer Care Plus, Duke Cancer Institute Wake County

Holly has delivered a beautiful, emotional tribute to her son Derek (a soldier) as he faced his toughest battle, with brain cancer. While specific to brain tumors, caregivers to patients of other life-threatening diseases can relate to the rollercoaster journey that faces many families navigating the health care system. The book is also filled with many helpful resources and shares the consoling words of fellow community members that rallied to support Holly and her family.

David Arons, Chief Executive Officer of the National Brain Tumor Society

One Hundred and Twenty-Six Days

The Unthinkable Journey

One Hundred and Twenty-Six Days

The Unthinkable Journey

Holly Richard

Holly Richard

ISBN: 978-1-944662-71-4

Publishing date: November 2021

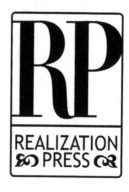

Cover Design by MASGraphics © 2021

Dedication

I dedicate this book to my precious son Derek, my amazing daughter Nicole, my best friend and husband Dave, and the countless other courageous and tenacious heroes who fought on this battlefield for Derek and with our family. I also dedicate this book to those precious lives who came before us and those who will come after us. I hope this book moves the reader and amplifies our agonizing pain until its sound is deafening and laser focused on annihilating and burying this beast once and for all.

Contents

Foreword

One Hundred and Twenty-Six Days is a story of the extraordinary bravery of Derek, his mother Holly Richard, and their family and others who walk this same path. This book is a deeply emotional, nonfiction account which allows the reader to share hope and agony along the way. This memoir offers the reader a rare opportunity to accompany family and friends on this unthinkable journey.

In this book, the author, Holly Richard, shares an incredible journey with the reader. The first section of the story begins in the present as we walk through the beginning of the unimaginable path with her. At a critical juncture, the story becomes reflective as the author looks back on events and shares insights and a deeper self-examination of the experience. In the last section, she looks forward and offers guidance and comfort for others who might also find themselves walking this winding trail.

I have intentionally kept this description vague so as not to dilute Holly's narrative. Sharing in the publication of this important book has been an honor, and I hope that after experiencing the journey, you are enriched and have a greater understanding of others who have confronted this challenge with courage and resilience.

Drew Becker
Publisher

TODAY

Chapter 1
Early December

Derek is super stoked about starting his next chapter in life! He's out of the Army and ready to turn the page. For nine years, he has been serving our country as a badass sky soldier in the 82nd Airborne. As a veteran traveler, the travel bug has gotten him again, and even though he is just home, he is looking for his next adventure. What healthy, adrenaline pumping 27-year-old soldier who jumps out of airplanes doesn't want to keep going, living life in the fast lane?

A few months prior to Derek coming home from the Army, he starts obsessing about cars. The only car he ever had was the one I gave him, my Ford Escape, and I had just paid off the loan, so it was a nice freebee. Over the six years he was stationed at Ft. Bragg, Derek needed a vehicle to drive back and forth to see his family. This momma (also known as "da momma") needed to see my son whenever possible, so the decision was pretty simple, and he was deeply grateful.

From his barracks in Italy, he's bombarding me with texts of numerous pictures of different cars until he finally finds his baby, a black and white Jaguar F-Type 150 two-door convertible, at a dealership in Texas. As soon as he arrives home from the Army, he is online figuring out how to do his first-ever purchase of anything other than food and necessities. Being single and living in Army barracks in a box for nine years, Derek didn't need a lot other than for his travel and music equipment.

Derek completes the application online for the purchase, and, when it's time to get the loan approved, I will never forget it (and I was waiting for that moment), he comes downstairs and gives me that "you are the best momma in the world" look followed by the "ask."

"Uh, da momma, so it looks as though I can't get the loan for the car unless you co-sign for me. You know I will make my payments and…"

I stop him quickly to save him from unnecessary begging.

"Derek, of course I will co-sign for you. I am so proud of you, I love you, you deserve that badass car, *and* I want to be the first to drive it—after you, of course!!"

He gives me that smile that boys give their momma and a hug I wish I could capture in a paper bag so I could let it out like a genie in a bottle whenever I need his hug. The flatbed truck arrives and delivers this badass car to our house. How crazy exciting! And let's just say this 27-year-old sky soldier turned back into that big brown-eyed seven-year-old little boy waiting for Santa to come down the chimney.

Derek looks forward to traveling to New York with a couple of Army buddies in December to see the ball drop on New Year's Eve. He has always found traveling exhilarating, but music feeds his soul. He had a DJing gig in Croatia while stationed in Italy; he has taught himself to make several songs thus far and has thousands of followers on Instagram. He is now laser focused on perfecting his music so he can share it with the world.

But first he goes with me and his stepdad, Dave, on a road trip to Georgia right after Thanksgiving to an open house at Atlanta Institute for Music and Media (AIMM). He enrolls in AIMM's two-year college program for Post Audio Production with his GI bill, and his first day of classes will be on January 7, 2019. We find a great apartment just a few minutes away, and there is also a Jaguar dealership nearby, which is the icing on the cake. We go to Rooms To Go with his sister Nic and order some really nice furniture for his new apartment. He is ready!

In early December, all of us go to pick out the Christmas tree and decorate it while playing Elvis Christmas songs, our family tradition. The house is so cozy, the fireplace is on, and the smell of a fresh-cut pine tree brings me back to when Nic and Derek were little. One Christmas when Derek was only three, he realized everyone gave me a present but him. He ran to his room, took one of his favorite hot wheel cars, wrapped it up in balled up wrapping paper, and gave it to me for my present. It was so precious! Santa gave him a football uniform and helmet for Christmas that year, and I couldn't get it off of him for days.

Derek is not feeling well. We assume it is just the winter cold. Then headaches start along with earaches, so we go to Urgent Care.

After he gets seen, the nurse practitioner approaches us.

"It is a sinus infection," she says.

That is good news, so off we go to Walgreens to fill the antibiotic prescription. In a few days, Derek says he is starting to feel better. He sends me a picture of the box of Ritz crackers and chicken noodle soup I left for him before I headed to work and his "Duv da momma" text. He always calls me "da momma" because I am *his* momma.

The morning of December 12, as I get ready for work, I hear the creaking floors as Derek walks upstairs.

In his tired voice, he says, "Mom, something is wrong. My head is killing me, and I just threw up."

"Oh, God, sweetie, that's not good. Let's get you to the hospital to find out what is going on."

Derek dresses, grabs his Gucci wallet, and gets in the car. I grab a puke bag and speed out of the driveway like a bat out of hell to the emergency room at WakeMed North.

On arrival, I notice the emergency room is empty, which is good. Derek shows his insurance card and ID, and we are immediately taken back to a room. Derek sits on the table, and I take a seat next to him.

"This must be a really bad sinus infection, D (I often call him D), and maybe mixed in with the flu. I am *so* relieved this place is empty, and we got right in," I say, keeping the talking light as his head is hurting so badly.

"Me too," he replies. "I feel like complete shit, Mom," he adds as he pukes in the bag.

"I guess you do! We are at the right place, D, and I am sure whatever you have, they will give you something."

The physician's assistant (PA) knocks at the door.

"Good morning," she says. "I am so sorry you are feeling so badly. Let's take a look and see what we can do to get you feeling better. What symptoms are you having, Derek?"

"I feel really bad," he says sounding exhausted. "I am having awful headaches and started throwing up this morning."

The PA continues to ask more questions to find out the culprit.

"How long has this been going on?"

I can read Derek's facial expressions, and I know my baby is in a lot of pain just trying to think and process the questions; he is exhausted and seems disoriented.

I take over. "It started a few days ago. I took him to Urgent Care, and they diagnosed him with a sinus infection. He started to feel better after taking the antibiotics for a few days. Then the other day, he said his headaches were back and getting worse, but it's weird because the headaches went away later in the day. Then Derek started throwing up this morning, and here we are. Thank goodness we didn't have to wait to see you!"

The PA is a gentle giant of a lady. As she looks over my son with such kind eyes, I know she will figure out what's going on so Derek can start feeling better. Christmas is only two weeks away, and the lucky duck is going to NY to watch the ball drop with his Army buddies. She keeps asking questions like what pharmacy do we use, are you allergic to any medicines, has Derek had these symptoms before, all the normal "why do you feel like shit" kinds of questions.

The PA says, "Derek, I think you do have a really bad sinus infection. But because you are throwing up, we are going to do a CAT scan just to be sure everything else looks okay."

The nurse assistant takes Derek down the hall for the CAT scan, and I am alone in the hospital room. I start texting Nic, letting her know we are at the hospital because Derek is feeling worse and throwing up.

Nic texts me back: "Mom, he *is* going to be okay, right?"

"Of course, he is, sweetie. I bet he has a dose of both a sinus infection and the flu combined!"

"Okay, good; text me as soon as you hear back."

"I will, sweetie."

I text Dave, my husband and my kids' stepdad, whom I also refer to as DJ (David Joseph), and at times he calls me HJ (Holly Jane). When we fell in love, DJ and HJ became one of the loving ways we referred to each other. I am texting Dave the same thing as Nic. I hit the send button and Dave calls me immediately.

Dave says, "I was leaving the house this morning, and Derek was up and said he felt like crap. I had no idea he was feeling that bad to go to the hospital!"

"It is okay. After you left, I went into the kitchen to make a cup of coffee, and Derek was coming out of the upstairs bathroom; he had just thrown up, so we hopped in the car and here we are. I am sure they will figure this out. The poor kid. I can tell he is feeling really crappy. I will text you once the tests come back."

"Okay, HJ. I love you."

"Love you too, DJ."

A few minutes later, Derek comes back to the room and pukes again in the new bag I put in the waste basket.

The PA comes in and I am sitting next to Derek with the wastebasket nearby. She and I lock eyes, those momma eyes that look scared to death, but you try to bluff so you can comfort your children when they are hurting, when they need boo-boos kissed, or they are afraid. She sits down, gently placing her hand on my knee.

"Derek, I am sorry to say that you have a large mass on the left side of your brain. We need to send you to the big WakeMed via an ambulance so we can monitor you throughout the trip."

Derek and I look at each other in disbelief. We can't comprehend what she is saying. How could this be? What could that be? I hug him so tightly, and he hugs me back harder. I call

Dave and Nic, who arrive in a matter of minutes. Next thing we know, Derek is on his way via ambulance and is admitted to the hospital on this chaotic and confusing morning of December 12, 2018.

Two consults from two different neurosurgeons and several MRIs and CAT scans later reveal a large tumor on the left temporal lobe of the brain. It is not only causing severe headaches and projectile vomiting, but it is affecting Derek's ability to think clearly or remember why he is even in the hospital. It needs to come out. A PET scan is done, and there are no other masses in other parts in his body. Otherwise, a biopsy would be needed to help identify what else might be going on and determine if this might be a type of cancer that could spread. The last thing you want to do is operate in the brain before ruling out all other options.

Derek is scheduled for brain surgery to remove the tumor on December 14. The hope is for a few days in the hospital followed by outpatient radiation and chemo at the Preston Robert Tisch Brain Tumor Center at Duke Hospital.

We wait for hours; I think it has been at least six-eight hours. All I know is it feels like years. The hospital is great about communicating with us via the hospital phone in the waiting area, giving us updates as they have them.

After the surgery, the surgeon comes out and says Derek did great. They were able to remove most of the tumor, and it came out quite easily like goo.

He continues, "We will biopsy the tumor to be sure we know what we are dealing with and get the results as soon as we can. We will also be in communication with the doctors at Duke Hospital where Derek will be getting his treatment. If all goes well here, he should be able to go home in a few days."

We all feel so relieved. Home in a few days—hallelujah!!!

Shortly after this, a nurse enters the waiting room.

"Derek did well, and he is in the recovery room. We will keep him there for a bit and then take him to the ICU to be monitored. Once he is moved to the ICU, we will let you know so you can see him."

"I want to see him now, please," I say, my voice quivering.

The nurse says, "I don't think that's a good idea; he is still coming out of the anesthesia."

I muster the strength to belt out, "I don't care. I want to see my son!"

Walking down the cold, white hallway, I try to prepare myself for what I will see. There he is, lying in a hospital bed, a half-shaved head revealing a horseshoe incision with at least 10 staples. I look into Derek's eyes; they are open, and the beautiful brown color in his eyes is gone. Instead, his eyes are black, all pupils, like staring into darkness. He thrashes his head back and forth like he is watching the ancient video game Pong. The nurse can see the terror in my eyes.

"It's okay, Mrs. Richard," she says. "It's normal, and he still needs more time in the recovery room."

I kiss Derek's right cheek and whisper in his ear, "Mom is here, sweetie, and I will be with you every step of the way."

Walking back through the cold, white halls, I keep it together as I know Derek's sister Nic will be staring into my eyes, searching for the same comforting expression that I was looking for two days ago in the emergency room with Derek. I adjust my gaze as I make my way back to the waiting area.

"Nic, D is doing okay. It is too early to see him though. He still has to come out more from the anesthesia after being under so long."

Nic, who is a chip off the ole block, demands to see him. I watch as she is escorted down the hall and again feel like I am going to hurl right there. I wait. She returns after a few minutes and collapses into my arms. We cry a river.

Chapter 2
Dazed and Confused

Derek doesn't come home in a few days as we had hoped. The tumor is in a really bad place. There are different areas of the brain that can give clues about what may be to come, and Derek's brain tumor is located where all the hard wiring for speech and mobility is. The surgery left Derek's right side completely immobile, and he has aphasia (also called word salad), which affects the production or comprehension of speech and the ability to read or write. He spends two weeks in the ICU and is starting to progress to where he does not need 24/7 nursing supervision and is moved to the step-down unit floor.

Nic and I cook Christmas dinner on Christmas Eve after a long day and night at the hospital. My amazing husband Dave, loving Dave, stays with Derek while his sister Nic and I go home and bring back all the fixings to the hospital and have Christmas dinner in Derek's room. We open presents and make the best of it. At the end of Christmas Day, Derek is finally medically cleared to move to WakeMed's inpatient rehab floor on December 26.

Once on the rehab floor, Derek is showing progress! His occupational therapist (OT) and physical therapist (PT) are able to get the muscles on the right side firing back up, and he is able to do leg presses with his right leg. Nic and I are so excited we take turns being in the therapy each day and video his progress as we cheer him on. He gradually is able to stand with two feet on the ground, holding onto the parallel bars and making a couple steps forward. We are so happy and take more video! Derek continues getting his strength back and can transfer from his wheelchair to his bed; he is making great strides. Working with the speech therapist is helping Derek to read and write again. We are sure in another three weeks he will be able to come home. Then he will start his six-week radiation/chemo outpatient plan at Duke to kill this tumor once and for all.

But that doesn't happen either. Shortly after New Year's, I can tell Derek is *off*. I can't describe it other than to say I know something is wrong. I ask for an MRI to be done, and they schedule it for the morning. At about four a.m. on January 4, the nurse calls me to tell me Derek has started vomiting. She thinks he is okay but wanted to let me know. My heart rises into my throat as I listen to her words. Vomiting means swelling in the brain; vomiting means hydrocephalus; vomiting means more fucking brain tumors!

I yell into the phone, "Please, God in Heaven, get the MRI done now, please, please, please."

I throw my clothes on and drive to the hospital. After I arrive in his room, he and his bed are gone, and I collapse on the floor. I look around the room and see one of his shoes on one side of the room and the other shoe across the room like people came flying in and out of there to get him for that MRI.

For those who have had an MRI of your upper body, you know it can be scary and claustrophobic and can make a brave person feel panicked. Can you imagine what Derek must be feeling? He just had brain surgery. Just a couple weeks ago he was riding around in his Jaguar, getting ready for the trip to New York to watch the ball drop and then moving to Georgia to start college. Now he is in this monstrous tube with deafening beeps as this machine scans for tumors. One day he is fine and the next he is living this horror movie, and we are all in it. What could be going through his mind? I feel like I will pass out.

They manage to finish the MRI, which produces more devastating news: fluid is building up on the brain, and the tumor has spread to other parts of his brain. Dear God, how can this be possible? Between the amazing collaboration of WakeMed and Duke, we can get Derek admitted to Preston Robert Tisch Brain Tumor Center at Duke in the evening.

While we are at Duke, several white coats are around Derek in his room, and I am so grateful so many eyes are on him. Derek starts screaming, "Mom, Mom, Mom" over and over again, and he passes out.

I am by his side telling him to hold on; I never felt so petrified in all my life.

I am grabbing and holding on to any white coat in my view, screaming and crying, "*What is happening to my son?*"

It is still January 4, 2019, and the radiation oncologist cannot start six weeks of radiation to fight these what the fuck (WTF) tumors until the doctors can keep the hydrocephalus (fluid in his brain) from building up. We find out that radiation is the only treatment option for his type of tumor, Glioblastoma grade IV, the Tumorator of all tumors. So for the next three days, the docs and nurses drain the fluid by the way of a lumbar drain, where they put a needle with a tube in Derek's lumbar spine to drain some of the cerebrospinal fluid (CSF) that fills the ventricles of the brain and surrounds the brain and the spinal cord.

More devastating news: these tumors are now able to travel via these ventricles and take the tumors to Derek's spine. Now Derek is experiencing excruciating headaches along with excruciating back pain, leg pain, nerve pain, and every God damn pain! He is now completely paralyzed on his right side again and unable to move anything much other than his left arm or his head.

After three days of draining the fluid, Derek's head pain is better. However, his radiation treatments cannot start if the fluid builds back up. Getting his head and spine blasted with radiation for six weeks can cause more fluid to build up, especially once the radiation starts killing off the tumors. The medical team will not let that happen. Therefore, they recommend another brain surgery to install a shunt in Derek's head that will push the fluid down and out of his brain and into his abdomen to prevent fluid from building back up.

Another important issue his medical team must consider is that Derek cannot have any open wounds on his body for about six weeks after radiation treatments start. The reason is twofold. The doctors will administer Avastin fusions right after radiation treatments are finished. Avastin is given to patients like Derek who have these WTF tumors, so Avastin can kill off any remaining tumors and hopefully keep more tumors from growing. However, the doctors will not administer Avastin if there are any open wounds on the body because it can compromise the immune system, the body's healing mechanisms, and can cause infections within the body. That means once radiation starts, Derek cannot have any more surgeries and this "one-two punch" is all we have with radiation to follow immediately by Avastin. It is our only hope. Derek does well with the second brain surgery to install a shunt, and now he is scheduled for six weeks of radiation.

Chapter 3
Radiation and the Mask

I receive Derek's radiation schedule and see that his thirty radiation treatments scheduled over the next six weeks are all over the map in terms of times each day. Some are in the morning and some in the afternoon. I immediately call the radiation department to change all of the appointments so they are every morning at 10:00 a.m. Thankfully they are able to reschedule them. That way, Derek can hopefully understand and adjust better to a schedule, and the nurses and I can learn the right medication regimen so we can make the radiation treatments bearable for him.

Two days into the radiation treatments, we get more devastating news. Derek needs another brain surgery to replace the valve in the shunt with a new low-pressure valve. (You can't make this stuff up—right out of a horror movie!) The radiation kills the tumor cells, but the tumor cells make the Cerebrospinal fluid (CSF) so thick that it clogs up the shunt. Then Derek is back to where the CSF builds back up on his brain, which causes excruciating head pain. He cannot continue to have surgery every time the fluid builds up. These tumors are so aggressive, and radiation has to continue. It is our only hope, so another brain surgery is scheduled, and the low-pressure valve is installed.

On January 12, 2019, at seven p.m., I wait for the nurses' shift change so I can be sure events of Derek's day, his meds, and all the communication are passed along to the night nurse. The nurses are so amazing. Although I am not a nurse, I know my child better than anyone. I can tell Derek's headaches are starting again. He is becoming quiet, non-responsive to my voice. The left side of his nostril begins to bother him every time fluid builds up in his brain; it starts messing with him up that left nostril. That means more swelling on the brain, more buildup of fluid, more fear, and panic about more pain. I stay and wait.

Derek's headaches are worsening. Medications and steroids aren't cutting it. Derek starts to moan, and then he starts yelling. Thank God for the God doctor! He is the neurosurgeon who installed the shunt and then did the second brain surgery to install the shunt with a low-pressure valve. He also installed a little button on the top of the shunt on Derek's head. The residency doctor came in once every hour throughout the night, pumping that button several times, which pushed the fluid off the brain. Derek is able to fall asleep, and each hour the residency doc quietly and patiently comes in all night long, pumping that button as Derek sleeps.

It is Tuesday morning, January 15, 34 days into this battle. Derek is fighting like a warrior. He is also struggling with wanting to let go and wanting to fight. His body is fragile now with little movement. He has lost over twenty pounds. Last month he was 150 pounds and now he looks so thin. His alertness is different; he is not himself. But the right regimen of medications to manage his pain allows him the ability to think without pain, and you can tell Derek is there. We are approaching the cancer crossroads as to where we go from here. What can the doctors continue to do? What does Derek want to do? Derek asked for help several times yesterday by saying help a few times, but he cannot find the words to tell us how we can help. Luis, our chaplain, gentle, patient, waiting in the corners and ready to appear like magic, is there to hear Derek's cries for help.

We all hold hands; I am holding Derek's left hand, the only limb with any life to it; he and I are both lefties. Luis says a prayer and we all finish the prayer with an "Amen."

Derek says, "5, 4, 3, 2, 1, let's do this," with a thumbs up and a grin. Derek is ready to continue with his radiation treatments, the only regimen available for his type of brain cancer.

As I sit quietly next to my son while he rests peacefully, I think back to all those hugs and kisses I took for granted. I think of his years of service to our country and how brave he was to enlist in the Army at 18 years old when he did boot camp at Fort Sill, Oklahoma. He was having a hard time adjusting to boot camp and wrote me letters every day he could. I remember how much he missed his candy. That kid loves all kinds of candy: Swedish Fish, Skittles, Reese's cups, sour gummy worms, Starbursts, Jelly Belly jellybeans, Junior Mints—you name it. When I would go to the grocery store, I always picked him up some sort of candy he liked because he liked them all. He would give me a hug and say, "I duv the momma." While he was at boot camp, he was really missing his candy, but the only way I could send him some was if I sent the entire troop candy. Bring it on! I went shopping, spent over $300.00 on candy, and shipped a big box to him and the troops. Derek was so appreciative; he had every soldier sign a thank you note to me.

Then on he went to Ft. Gordon and studied to become a signal system support specialist. From there he went to Ft. Benning for 82nd Airborne training. I had the biggest honor of all; I pinned my son's airborne wings onto his uniform at graduation, one of my most precious memories. I think of how he navigated his way to 25 countries in less than three years while stationed in Italy and how he put these experiences into the self-taught music he made. Then his determination to enroll in college after serving nine years in the Army. His life as we knew it has been taken from him, stripped from him in an instant.

Cancer is taking over his once strong body, and I've never felt so helpless in my life. The pain and heartache are overwhelming. I feel I cannot breathe sometimes. Other times I feel I could kill something. The beast comes charging out of the cave, anything to punch, to claw at, to relieve my rage as I watch my son fight for his life, a life he so deserves to live. Why this, why Derek, why, why, why????

It's still Tuesday in the late morning when we arrive back to the room from the fourth radiation treatment. I want to climb into his bed with him and listen to his heartbeat and cradle him, to kiss the top of his head as I did so many years ago. But there are so many tubes, and he's losing more weight. His body is so thin, and his spine has painful tumors, so I lean in and lay my head next to his on his pillow and feel his breath on my face. Many times since we have been living in the hospital I have been told that where there is life, there is hope. We have hope and we *will* be getting out of the hospital and home to our new life soon.

Regardless of the meds Derek is given prior to radiation, he still awakens in that mask with his frail body strapped to the table, unable to move until the radiation targets and destroys the tumors. I can only imagine what that must feel like. Probably like being in a horror movie. Now the anxiety levels and stress escalate for me. I fear the dead tumor cells will clog the shunt; then the fluid will back up and put pressure again on his brain, causing more savage pain. The doctors come in every hour and pump the little button on the top of his head to push down the fluid. Do we do another surgery to unclog it and keep going?

How much can Derek stand of that, going under each time, anesthesia, breathing tube, then recovery period? Then back to the radiation table again. I have to sign one form after another to approve these treatments. My God, why is this happening to my precious son?

It is January 16, 2019, 5:30 a.m. I desperately need sleep but can't nod off. I get ready and arrive at Duke at 6:30 a.m. It is raining and so dark and cold outside. I am relieved to snag a good parking space on the first floor of the parking garage. I am in the elevator and trying to prepare for whatever the day holds for Derek. The elevator sounds its bell, and I make my way down the corridor filled with windows wrapped in the darkness of the morning. The nurse at the front window looks at me and gives a gentle smile. No need to ask me who I am or to show ID; I am a regular here now. She pushes the button to release the lock so I can make my way to the hallway that leads to Derek's room.

As I approach his hall, the nurses are gathered at the nursing station, sharing their information about their patients for shift change. Many look up and greet me with their soft smiles and eyes of sympathy and love for Derek and our family. As I enter his room, I slowly pull the hospital curtain back, trying to be as quiet as possible in case he is still sleeping. I slowly make my way to Derek's bed when, all of a sudden, he thrusts his head forward as far as it will go with strength that I have not seen since he's been in the hospital, leaving his torso, arms and legs lifeless on the bed, and screams:

"Mom, I want to die; please let me *die!*" Derek slams his head back onto the pillow and starts to sob. I start to dry heave but manage to curb it since I haven't eaten much in the past couple days. My insides are vibrating, my whole body starts shaking, and my legs are barely holding me up. What do I say?

"Derek, I am so sorry you are having to go through this living hell. I do know that we all agreed that you are 27 years old and your heart, lungs, and organs are all healthy. You are disciplined from your years in the Army, and the docs are hopeful you will be one of the lucky few. We just have to get through the six weeks of radiation, and you will have a chance to beat this and come home, but this is the only way; this is the only treatment option you have. Please, D, please keep trying."

His crying stops, he stares at the ceiling for several minutes and then turns to me. We lock eyes and share another moment in the hospital where there are no more words to be spoken in the cold, dark hours of the morning.

It is January 17, 2019, 7 a.m. Derek had a good day yesterday, which means we were able to manage pain, and he is alert and able to communicate with a lot of talking, even though much of it was word salad, and some of his personality is in full gear. This morning, he looks so much like himself and is resting comfortably. Each morning I arrive with my stomach in my throat and my heart pounding as I wonder what kind of day he and I are facing. Thirty-six days into this new world, I try so hard to let go of the selfishness of keeping him here with us, here on this earth, and try to accept that his life is in God's hands.

I am so angry at God and now doubt that there is even a God. I cannot imagine my life without my son in it. Yet I know all too well from my 20+ years as a service provider in nonprofits about quality of life and what that means. It is certainly not this hell he is living in since early December.

Derek is lethargic when he wakes up. He perks up some and then starts throwing up quite a bit. I get the nurse acquainted with Derek's pain meds regimen before radiation, and I also ask if we can start nausea medications for the next couple days. Radiation is probably the most stressful time of the day for me because

I know it is for Derek. Derek stares at his right arm, tattooed with a full sleeve, the arm that has been paralyzed since the first surgery. The arm is much thinner now. Derek takes his left hand and lifts his right arm, he stares at it more, then drops the right arm, and it flops back down on the bed. He looks at me. I try to say comforting words and to give him hope. Then he stares back at me, slowly turns his head left to right, making a "stop it" gesture. His eyes fill up with tears, and he stares out the window where the world once was.

It is 2:00 p.m. For the first time, Derek did well on the radiation table; the pain med regimen is working, I think. No moving and no expletives, so those are good signs. He loves the Chick-fil-A peach shakes I greet him with right after his treatments. His eyes go wide, and it is like he has been in the desert for days without food or water. He sucks on the straw as the transportation staff takes him, his bed, and me through the labyrinth of hallways to get us back to his room on the eighth floor.

He is resting now. I start researching on my laptop to see what VA benefits may be available to him. I pray he not only wins this battle but he is able to come home and live a good life, and I want him to have the money and resources to do so. After nine years of service, he deserves whatever is available to him as a veteran.

It is Sunday, January 20, at 7 a.m. Three days later feels like three years of being on constant guard. Derek had more vomiting on the 18th, so he has nothing by mouth for now. We have to come up with another pain management plan since he was taking most of his medications by mouth. He enjoyed visitors, his buddies from Waynesville, yesterday.

Derek is quiet this Sunday morning. When I tried to hold his hand to say good morning, he pulled his left hand away, letting me know that now was not the time. I can tell pressure is building in his head. The nurse comes in with scheduled pain meds, and he is now resting comfortably. Given the pain in his head and back, we are not sure how we can get him up. The pain becomes more intense when anyone tries to move him. We have been able to manage pain with little movement in the bed, but just getting him repositioned can cause great discomfort.

I am at a loss at what to do. I always can figure out something. I survived many painful and challenging events in my life. I have been able to take care of my children and support them through whatever life brings to them. This is by far the biggest mountain God has given me to climb. I am trying with all that I have, and Derek is too.

On January 21, Derek cannot keep any food down; his swallowing is weakening, and he is losing more weight. His doctors recommend a feeding tube. Jesus Christ, a feeding tube!! I lose my breath again followed by sheer panic and then shock. This means another surgery and feeding him liquid food poured into a tube in his stomach. My God! I know this all too well because of my work. I order a meeting for the following morning, and I demand the medical team is in attendance with the lead doctors, the social worker, and palliative care team—every hand on deck.

Dave, Nic, and I walk into the meeting and sit down. Derek's father, who lives in another state, calls in to the meeting and is on speaker phone. I am so grateful that everyone is there for Derek and our family. I discuss our concerns about how much further we go with his treatment. We then talk about survival rate for people with glioblastoma (GBM), which is on average six to eighteen months. He has little quality of life; he is suffering and the reality of what this cancer does and is doing to Derek and its wrath continues to be unthinkable. We then went back in time to our conversations in early January that we had with Derek and our family, where we all agreed we had to get the six weeks of radiation treatment finished for Derek to have a chance. Again, as they say a lot at this hospital, where there is life, there is hope. At the time of those conversations, Derek was cognizant enough to understand the treatment was going to be really hard, and he would feel like total crap for most of that time.

We discussed again that the radiation (followed by several infusions of Avastin) is the *only* treatment option for this type of horrific Tumorator. And the only way Avastin can be safely administered is if there are no open wounds in the body for at least four to six weeks. As mentioned earlier, Avastin keeps the body from being able to fight off infections. We agreed this was going to be six weeks of hell.

The team once again reminds all of us that Derek is young, healthy, and disciplined. We all hope Derek and the medical team can fight this Goliath. I know the feeding tube will provide nutrition and is the only way we can manage his pain going forward. It is the only way he will survive the next few weeks of treatment. Where there is life, there is hope, so once again I sign the papers for the surgery.

I find myself observing young couples with children walking by our rooms as they make their way to the to the hospital's waiting areas. My heart aches once again, knowing that for Derek life is so uncertain. Survival feels like it is hour by hour sometimes. I watch helplessly every day now as Derek views the nurse pour his meals into the feeding tube. I can read his facial expressions; he is unable to process what is happening. He looks confused as he focuses on the blue gloves pouring liquid into his stomach. His eyes are squinting in disbelief that he is really seeing what he is seeing. Then he looks up at the ceiling. Another punch to our guts.

Food is Derek's number one satisfaction. Life's race took him to 25 countries, traveling around the globe and eating fish and chips in London, sitting on London Bridge, sushi in Japan and Belgian waffles in Belgium. He took me with him on his magic carpet ride via FaceTime where he was riding camels in Egypt, dabbing at the Great Wall of China, touring Stonehenge, zip lining down the tallest building in Dubai, and having owls sit on his head in Japan. While he loves food, music is his passion. He made several songs and DJed in Croatia. Can you believe he made the cut for new artist and hopped over to Croatia to perform at the Ultra Europe Festival? He came home from the Army and enrolled in a college to master his music, to perfect it. And then this happens. How can this possibly be real?

I watch helplessly again as Derek has a bowel movement in his diaper. His facial expressions are communicating how disgusted he feels about it all. He now allows me to help him with his diaper when he has to pee. Peeing in the jug that hangs on the side of the hospital bed is the one thing he has been able to continue to do independently on a good day. This cancer sucks everything out of a person, right down to oneself, one's dignity. My heart aches for him, for us, for me. I begin to think how just weeks ago he was so healthy, full of life. The dreams I had hoped for him—to see a girl steal that loving heart of his, to have a family, grandchildren—it is all so distant now.

It's January 29, 2019, 8:45 p.m. I am eating dinner at home, looking for Derek still, miraculously, to come around the corner to greet me after a long day at work, just one more time, just once more. Instead, it is another long day at the hospital filled with so many emotions and also with people who have enormous hearts. So many come to see this young man at the hospital and how strong he is to go 12 rounds with this godforsaken cancer.

Derek has a day of rest from pain and handled radiation well this morning. He seems to know when I am alone with him. He looks at me like the soldier son he is to me, and he knows what he is facing. He has served nine years in the military, so he is used to taking orders and doing what he is ordered to do. However, I am mom, and there is this ever-peaceful sharing that we do, just the two of us, where he knows I am fighting right beside him, I am listening to what he struggles to say, that this is really tough stuff. I hear him via his soul, and he hears me through mine. Forty-eight days later, here we are. WTF?!

My daughter Nic is such an incredible sister and loves her brother more than anything. My husband Dave has taken both my children under his wing as I do Dylan, Dave's son, my stepson, and we really do have three children together. There has been so much love and support, so many tears and tough times spent at the hospitals these past couple months, and Derek knows he is not alone in this fight. We are all family strong. Somehow, though, I go back to writing just about him and me. Because that is where I spend each and every day—with Derek. I do not know what the MRI will show in the next few days. Is the treatment working? If so, what does that mean when you have incurable cancer? What does life after Duke even look like? If we even get to that point, what would Derek want? My everyday prayer is for Derek to recover and be restored to the healthy and happy life he had before this ruthless cancer started to devour his being. If that can't be, then I pray for Derek to be able to take the wheel and travel to the destiny of his choice.

On February 5, I look at Derek's large communications/erase board in the hospital room. Being in the hospital over time has a way of making everything upside down. I feel like I am sitting on the ceiling, and the floor is above my head. I cannot remember where my car is parked in the hospital garage anymore and walk aimlessly at night like a zombie trying to locate it. Sometimes I have to go find the security guard in the parking garage to help me search for it in his golf cart. I take pictures now with my cell phone of signage and landmarks so I can look back at them in the evening and can find my way back to my car to drive myself home somehow.

I am not sure what day it is nor what time other than when radiation is and when the transportation team comes to take Derek and his bed. I am with him every day as we go to radiation, holding the side of the bed and ensuring we go slowly over uneven floor surfaces and never to let the bed bump the wall as we navigate through the many hallways and elevators to get to radiology. The smallest movement can send knife-stabbing pain into Derek's body. I also know when OT/PT/SLP may stop by and that the lift team comes every two hours to re-position Derek the best they can without causing further pain for him. I know the schedules of the nurses and assistants who have kept him so clean and well cared for and other people that are important in Derek's care like the kitchen staff, dietician, and housekeeping. It takes a village to care for a person with a brain tumor.

We were given a glimmer of hope from doctors yesterday morning. The MRI reveals shrinking tumors; they are not multiplying elsewhere like little gremlins; they are shrinking! Of course, the cancer is incurable, cells will keep mutating, and does that even make sense? Right now, we are one step closer to Derek feeling better. His pain is also so much better and pain meds are now IV Dilaudid every one-two hours and oxycodone every three hours and fentanyl patches along with IV Tylenol. And who knew there was such a thing as liquid caffeine that helps with head pain that we could administer intravenously? All of this just to get him up in hopes that he can sit in a wheelchair without painful headaches.

I sit and look at the bag of liquid food, the anti-nausea meds, steroids, bowel movement meds, and lotion to keep his feet soft—it is incredible. I keep asking how this happened to my son. How can this just be bad luck? One day a gene stops producing proteins. Cells in your body decide that today is the day that when the cells start to divide without the exact DNA like they once were every second of every day for the past 27 years of Derek's life. All of a sudden, an initial molecule event happens in one cell that sets the process of becoming an actual cancer in motion event. Really?! Then additional sequential mutations take place within the tumor cell's DNA and gain the ability to grow uncontrollably and invade healthy tissues like little demons. Then they start killing him, and this is one big molecular clusterfuck, and no one knows why, so they refer to it as "bad luck." Are you kidding me, people?! But it is real, so painfully real.

Radiation treatments have been going well over the past two weeks. After the first week of hell, we were able to work out the medication regimen between nursing and radiology so Derek would be okay when strapped in the iron maiden mask, a mask they made specifically for him to begin radiation. The mask is so tight that it leaves all of these small, dotted imprints on his face and head that fade away within an hour. The mask is webbed. I cannot think of words to describe it as I have nothing to reference other than like a chain linked fence smashed up against your face. It has to be iron clad tight because one move and radiation could hit a spot that could be dangerous, or they would have to start over again. And 30-35 minutes in that mask, strapped on to a skinny, hard, pull-out drawer with eight-inch Velcro straps over your chest and legs is more than the mind can grasp. It is too large to think it. The med regimen is helping more now to be sure he doesn't wake up while he is strapped down wearing the mask like he is in a Stephen King thriller. I have only seen the mask when the radiation therapist walks past us as we wait each morning for Derek to be taken to the back room. My mind can't begin to imagine it. This is too large of a nightmare to think about it. Until today.

Derek has been snoring most mornings as we wait in the back room of radiology for the technicians to come get him and wheel him and his bed to the radiation room. Snoring is a sign meds are in check, and it should be another calm and still time on the radiation table. As I wait in the waiting room, I begin pacing more. It seems like Derek has been in there too long. I continue to look for a radiation tech I know so I can find out what is happening. Then Nelson, the sweetest radiation therapist of all time with dark, kind eyes, appears and walks towards me. I study his eyes like never before. I am a social worker by trade, and I can read body language, I can interpret postures, and I can read eyes that are telling me something is wrong!

Nelson says, "We had to stop the treatment. Derek is moving around and swinging his left arm inside the radiation tube. We are trying to get another dose of Dilaudid pulled."

I know from Nelson's voice and his eyes that getting this treatment finished today is important.

Nelson asks, "Do you want to go to the radiation room and see if your voice can calm him?"

Oh, my God, I don't want to see that, my son with that mask on him, something I could only imagine until now. I think I might vomit. I suck in a big, bad wolf breath. "Yes, absolutely, where is he?"

Nelson guides me into the dark radiation room where green lights are randomly flickering, and there he is. Strapped in onto the board. The mask that has been horrific glimpsing it in passing is now strapped so tightly to Derek's head and shoulders. His hospital gown is off. I can see his chest rising and falling so fast.

The incisions on his head from multiple brain surgeries and his shunt tube and the feeding tube are all exposed. My eyes are on overload, and my heart is about to shatter into a million pieces. I am trying so hard to focus and to not pass out. I can hear Derek's faint whimpers through the mask. I suck in another massive breath and with all the momma strength I have, I whisper:

"Derek, it is Mom, and I am right here with you."

I walk to the other side of the tube so I can softly hold his left hand, the only limb on his body that moves, and cradle his hand in mine.

"It will only be a few more minutes more. Okay, sweetie, almost done."

Derek lets out a breath, the thrusting in his chest begins to slow down, his breathing settles, and he lays his left arm back down so they can re-Velcro and strap him back in. I leave the room and hold the wall. One of the radiation techs comes over and hugs me and thanks me.

"Sometimes, only a mother can do it. I know how hard that was," she says.

I have no words. I want to say no mother *should* ever have to do this. But I know she means well. I walk back out to the waiting room, my legs barely able to hold me up. I am in disbelief at what I saw. I am not sure if I am grateful for being at the brain tumor center of the world or cursed for being at the brain tumor center of the world.

When the radiation treatment finishes, the technician comes to get me. Derek lies in his bed in the wait area with tears in his eyes. I can read his eyes, and he is relieved it is over. The nurse gives Derek the Dilaudid that we hoped to have earlier, and she tears up too. This is another glimpse into a day in the life of someone with such aggressive brain cancer. Someone so beautiful, young, our son, Nic's brother. It is all so unfair he has to go through something so awful, so hard and traumatic. He should never be battling this cancer that came out of nowhere, yet here we are, the radiation techs, nurses, and all of us around Derek's bed, so angry at this cancer, and all of us loving Derek.

On February 5, I leave the hospital at 5 p.m. while it is still light outside. I usually stay 12-16 hours a day or as long as my mind and my body can last. Between Dave, Nic and me, we always wait for nursing shifts to change to be sure Derek's treatment regimen and the communication is carried from one shift to the next. I walk around the lake; it is 76 degrees from what I hear on the radio. My body needs the movement after so many long days sitting in the hospital. Again, my mind goes to my precious son, lying in the hospital bed in diapers, unable to move anything but his left arm. The air is warm; how I wish Derek was next to me. He and his sister and I walked beside this lake together a few times in the past, Derek on his skateboard mostly.

As I hike the winding trails, I am acutely aware, more than ever before, about all that is going on in my world right now. My awareness is overwhelming. My heart starts to ache badly again as I see moms with little sons. Their little boys ride their bikes with training wheels and decorated helmets, trying to go fast like Superman. The moms are nervous but trying to let them experience being a child on a bike. Then I see young families all together, and again my heart aches wishing my son could experience what true love in its purest form feels like from someone he can imagine living with for the rest of his life. And that beam of hope for a grandchild so I can look into their little eyes and see Derek's big brown eyes with those long fluttering eyelashes like butterfly wings. To feel his arms wrap around my neck like angel wings makes my heart ache so much I think it will just slide out of me. Derek surviving and having a quality of life for however long, that is enough, to hug him and know he is Derek.

My wonderful husband calls me on the way to the hospital after a grueling day in his Medicaid world. His voicemail sounds like it did before all this happened. "Hi, HJ; it's David Joseph." How I wish I could take myself back to those days when these phone calls were a sigh of relief that the long day at work was over. Instead, I dread going into the night where I have these recurring nightmares that I am sinking to the bottom of the sea. My lungs fill up with saltwater and choke me until I finally wake up. Why my precious boy? Why anyone's precious loved one; why?

As of February 7, 2019, there have been some noticeable improvements for Derek, meaning he's closer to hopefully more pain relief. Nourishment is good now with the feeding tube and less pain meds are needed. His bowels are working better to avoid the dreaded enemas, and, my God, please grant him the mental status and cognizance to be the captain of his own ship! We all agreed to the six-week radiation gauntlet, but no one could prepare for all the other unimaginable things happening. With the guidance of the doctors and the palliative care team, Nic, Dave, and I are at least seeing signs that Derek may have that opportunity to return to some sort of quality of life, which he so deserves. We are praying Duke can get Derek through the last radiation treatment on February 22. He has a convoy now of hands and hearts that are lifting him every time they see him. And Derek thanks them most days. Even when he is at his lowest, he still will almost always say thank you to his caregivers.

Yesterday afternoon was another heart stabbing time when Derek was so angry and so sad. Comforting him was impossible.

His heart rate skyrocketed, and the pain was everywhere. Although his words are not coming out in a way that is understood by one of his nurses, I understand Derek. I can read him so well even with brain tumors in his brain! He is watching me as I set up the iPad on his hospital table next to his bed. I am panicking and trying to get the iPad to work so maybe a movie or music would give him a snippet of relief. Perhaps I could find the Rick and Morty show with Pickle Rick, one of his favorite episodes. Anything that offers a reprieve from this living hell.

Suddenly, he slowly puts his hand on mine. Our eyes connect. I see his eyes and I immediately feel them stare into my soul, into my body that carried him in my womb for nine months, feeling his heart beating like I did 27 years ago. I am watching on the outside but feel I cannot reach him. I have had this tormented dream on several occasions where I am in a hospital gown and in Derek's bed. I am Derek and I am looking around and disoriented. I cannot move, my heart is racing, and I get so scared, but I get to wake up from the horror I was feeling in that dream. Derek is living it. He is trying to tell me in the only way he knows how that he knows what this cancer is doing to him. He sees me and his sister hurting, his eyes telling the whole story. He wants to leave and does not care what that means. Just get me out of this hospital, and if it is to leave this world, so be it.

I do not have the linguistic capacity to explain the utter helplessness of those ten minutes. The doctor orders Ativan, and within a couple minutes Derek looks at me with relief but also with sadness. My heart hurts more than ever. I kiss his cheek.

"I love you, D."

"I love you too, da momma."

"Do you want to watch a movie?"

"Okay," he says in a weak voice.

We find something he likes, the comedian Gabriel "Fluffy" Iglesias, and we begin watching. I realize it has been 12 hours at the hospital, and I am so tired, barely able to hold my weak body upright.

"Sweetie, I need to go home, and I will see you first thing in the morning. Okay?"

"Okay," he says as he turns to look at me.

I watch as his eyes find their way back to the iPad. I cry all the way to the car, and once inside I somehow find my cut-off valve deep within me, knowing that I desperately need to numb myself enough to get home safely. It is my emergency valve I created in my mind many years ago when I was a little girl starving to be loved by a mother and a father who didn't know how to give the kind of love I needed. Not sure which, but the hunger pangs for love are the same kind of pain. Love can be beautiful, and it can be painful. I learned early on how to survive. Being able to go numb for a period of time is survivor's mode. I feel at times I will not survive this heartache; the pain is unbearable. My mind wanders back to those beautiful brown eyes; Derek needs me more now than ever to get him where he wants to be. Whatever destiny he chooses, I must be there for him.

On the night of February 10, we managed to pull off Nic's 34th birthday celebration with some of our dearest friends. I was not sure how I was going to organize it all, but I did. We celebrated Nicole's birthday as best as we could. How deeply special she is to us and to the world. The guilt crept in at times as my mind raced back to Derek. How could we be out to eat while he is in the hospital? Seeing Nic's beautiful smile that I have not seen for weeks made it obvious why. She deserved a reprieve too from being the big sister watching her brother fight for his life. Nic was struggling with her own disease called "an eating disorder"

(ED) from hell. How I hate eating disorders and brain tumors, two totally different diseases. Why would I even put them in the same sentence? I guess it is because they both are depleting the life of my children, and I cannot kill these diseases; I cannot hurt them, nothing. I have to fight with all of my being every day with no sword, just my exposed heart. I know how terrified David felt staring up at Goliath.

Today is the best we have seen of Derek in weeks. I am convinced prayers work; at least today I believe. All around the world, prayers have been going on for Derek. There it is right in front of me—the power of prayer and that higher power I shut out of my soul so many moons ago. When I arrive this morning, pain consult docs are outside Derek's room. I start to walk faster in fear and then notice their casual discussions and laid-back stances in those white jackets. I walk in and Derek is tearful, so depressed, the doctor leaning over him, calming him, listening to my Derek like he has no other patients to see but my Derek. I say "hi" to Derek and kiss his cheek. He leaves the sad state he is in and soon after transitions to a better space. Derek spends the remainder of the day awing his sister and me with good receptive language and responses and eating half of his lunch! He is putting a few sentences together in conversations with four special young men and friends that came to visit with him. They are all laughing and talking Xbox talk. Derek is an avid gamer, and his friends tell me he is the best, and they always put him at the top of the team list. Their visit breathed energy into Derek's tired body and gave us all a sliver of normalcy and hope.

Chapter 4
Where There Is Life, There Is Hope...

So much can happen in a week, a day, in an hour, a minute when you are dealing with this relentless cancer. Derek finishes his six weeks of radiation which is a miracle in itself. Nelson, the radiation tech, asks Derek if he wants his radiation mask and Derek says yes. I look at that mask that passes by me each day as they carry it through the hall and into the radiation room and then strap it on him and shoot his brain and body with radiation. I hate that mask, which leaves marks from that wire basket embedded on his forehead, face, and shoulders. Now the mask sits there in Derek's hospital room, and I look at it differently. It saved his life—at least during the past six weeks. We still have Derek and that is hope.

Derek has been doing really well. His appetite is back, and his communication has improved. Although his speech is still word salad at times, he says that he loves me more often. I want a perfume like that, *my son loves me* perfume. The doctors at Duke clear Derek to transfer back to WakeMed on their neuro inpatient rehab this time. This is amazing and such a relief, but it also scares me. All the doctors and nurses know him here at

Duke; they understand the drill. Now I have to go through another boot camp of getting everyone on the same page, especially me. I now know how our families feel where I work, families that have children with disabilities, and I understand how they depend on our agency to support and love their child in our care 24 hours a day, seven days a week. The hopelessness is overwhelming. You want to trust those who are doing the job of caring for your child, yet *you* know what is best, or at least as parents we think that way.

Once again, I will have to train and educate the nurses shift by shift as well as the doctors and the on-call docs. They will need to know how to read Derek's cues, how you can tell when there is fluid building up on his brain or when he is getting constipated. I have to explain about the shooting pain all over his body that can happen just by gently repositioning him every two hours, changing and bathing him, anything. It is like working with paper-thin glassware. When it comes to meals, he can only eat with his left hand, so I'll have to tell them not put his tray on the right side of the bed. Since he can only move his left hand, he needs assistance cutting up food and managing how to eat it. I have never felt so tired. I can't be there all the time, yet I cannot trust that anyone else knows Derek better than me. Unless I am able to keep my eyes on Derek at all times, I struggle to do anything but stay in fear.

Unbeknownst to me and my husband, Derek purchased Elton John tickets back in October, two months before getting poisoned by tumors. He knows how much I love Elton and that I have never seen him in concert. Derek sat us down one evening in November and surprised us with tickets to the concert. This was his way of saying thank you for letting him live with us over the few months until he was due to move to Georgia to start college in January. What a thoughtful young man, my son. I gave him a big hug until he told me I could let him go. I was so excited and could not wait to see Elton belt out "B-B-B Bennie and the Jets."

Little did we know Derek would be in the hospital with brain cancer on March 12, 2019, the night of the concert.

When Dave and I find our seats, we can't believe how close we are! We are dead center of the stage, first row from the floor. OMG, these are amazing seats! Derek must have paid several hundred dollars for these tickets. Elton comes out and, sure enough, "Benny and the Jets" is the first song he plays. My heart races, and I sing from the top of my lungs word for word. The songs bring me back to my childhood years when music saved my soul. Music saved Derek's soul too until cancer picked him to prey on. I take pictures and videos to show Derek.

I told Derek the night before when I was leaving the hospital that we were going to the concert, and he gave me that lefty smile. By this time, Derek's right side of his face is paralyzed, so when he smiles it looks more like a half moon that starts from the corner of his left side of his lips all the way up to the bottom of his left eye. It is a big lefty grin, and anytime he smiles is a gift. The next morning, I can't wait to show Derek. I play him some of the video from the concert, and he looks at me with such a happy face and that big, half-moon smile. I felt his happiness at that moment, another gift he gave to me.

On March 26, 2019, I arrive home at 7:30 p.m. from a day at the hospital, reading a "Neuro Care Team Conference Report" about my son, our son, Nicole's brother. Never in a million years would I think I would be reading a treatment team's report on my child. "Simple Man," a song by Lynyrd Skynyrd, comes on, and I lose it for a minute. It was, after all, a song Derek played for me several years earlier, and he danced with me to that song at my wedding when I married Dave. That was the first time I had the honor to slow dance with my handsome soldier son since he became an adult. He gleefully accepted dancing with "da momma" in the living room as a child or even outside at the bottom of the mountain where we lived. He was a live wire, that child, and wore me out every chance he could!

The more I read this report, the more I want to hurt someone, especially because it was hand delivered to me at the end of the day in his room on Derek's 28th birthday. The social worker then turned to Derek to wish him a happy birthday and disappeared out of the room and down the hall.

The report says, "Discharge date 4/3/2019 to my home as there is no nursing home bed in a 50-mile radius and Derek will need 24/7 nursing services and personal care services."

Obviously the social worker is disconnected, maybe from her own workload, maybe from life. Maybe because she has had to deal with me, this crazy ass mom after 104 days in the hospital, watching my son fight, give up, and regain hope, tenacious, suffering, all the ugliness of an evil brain tumor. All of this while watching my precious daughter Nic fighting for her life too, dealing with her eating disorder (ED), also a ruthless, conniving demonic disease. The food that brings Derek the only comfort he can have brings Nicole her greatest fears. All of this insanity in the same room. It feels as though my head will cave in, and then I feel the rage of the beast. Its target is on anyone who dares to be in my view.

Later, thinking back on Derek's 28th birthday, it feels like a celebration for his sister and me. We ate Taco Bell and cookie cake with ice cream, and, of course, those Reese's eggs! When Nic and I had to leave, we hugged and cried with Derek. It was painful, yet it is what families do, and it felt for a moment abnormally normal. Then Nic and I had another cry, the bonding of a mother and child in the hospital hall as we said goodbye. Such a beautiful soul she is, so grateful to have her. She did save my life when she came into this world when I was barely 22 years old. That is a whole other book. She is amazing, everything about her.

Chapter 5
Washing Clothes

I remember when my kids were little, it seemed as though laundry was, at minimum, a daily chore. I often wondered how in the hell my Aunt Nancy managed to keep up with her nine children's clothes along with hers and my Uncle Fran. I remember vividly what the house looked like from top to bottom. It was my favorite place to be—other than when we vacationed in Maine with all of them, my Aunt Nancy, Uncle Fran, and all my cousins. I was so happy to be invited and it was my happy place. I was safe there. I was loved, and I had plenty of good food to eat. We kids would head out with our buckets and go clam digging for hours. My Uncle Fran would catch some crab and lobsters in his cages off his boat, and we had a feast of seafood right from the sea and all of it free.

I remember one day while on vacation in Maine, I watched my Aunt Nancy spend hours picking every sliver of crab out of every nook and cranny of those crabs with the tiny little forks. I remember it well because their dog Snoopy bit me in the face the night before when I bent down to pet him while he was eating—bad idea. Aunt Nancy wanted to be sure I was okay, so I had to stay back that day when all of my cousins headed out to the waters and adventures of the day. You would think I would have been so upset, but I wasn't. I craved to be loved like a mom loves her child, and Aunt Nancy gave me that love, maternal love, unconditionally. I could just feel it, and it was a feeling I never had felt before. As I watched her from the bed I was lying on next to the kitchen, she asked me how I was feeling and took the bandage off my eye to be sure it still looked okay. It was a close call. It could have been my eyeball he chomped on. Snoopy bit a lot of kids but not bad enough to make people too worried, so he stayed around; he was family too.

Walking into Aunt Nancy and Uncle Fran's home on Nelson Street in Grafton, Massachusetts, was for me walking into the best place in the world. They lived there for 63 years together and raised all nine children there. They both passed away within ten months of each other a few years ago. My cousin Lor, who is like my sister, is one of nine children, three girls and six boys. She and my other cousins carry so much grief. Her sister Cheryl passed away at age 37 many years ago followed by her sister Trisha at 58 years old, and just last year we lost Cousin Tommy at age 58 to cancer. It felt like I lost my very own sisters, brothers, and parents too.

Oh, and the aroma of Aunt Nancy's cooking and the fresh smell of Noxzema cream, the "heal all" cream. She slapped it on any bare skin she saw come past her. For some reason, many of my nine cousins, me included, would get leg aches as children. Our kneecaps started aching, and then our whole legs started hurting, and rubbing it with Noxzema made the aches go away. I have not heard of such a thing since becoming a parent, and I have never heard anyone say, "My child has leg aches."

No one entered the home from the front porch, and I believe because back then there were not stairs to step up to the front porch, so you would park on the side of the home or on the front lawn, depending on how many cars were there, and enter the home through the back door. Immediately to the right was a bathroom that had the only washing machine for eleven people, and next to it was always a mountain of dirty clothes. The clothes were hung out on a clothesline in the backyard. Like I said, how could you keep up with all the clothes?! Having that memory of the mountain of clothes that never disappeared, I was relieved that my pile of clothes was an anthill compared to the McClure's mountain of clothes. I would smile at times while putting Derek and Nic's clothes in my washing machine. Their little Ninja Turtle and Mickey Mouse pajamas, T-Rex, princesses and fairies, dinosaurs, and monster trucks—their clothes made me laugh and beam with pride at my two beautiful children who looked so much alike. My kiddos.

When Derek came home from the Army in April 2018, just a few months before he became sick, I began to notice his taste for expensive clothes. He traveled to some pretty amazing places, and I think he developed some of his high-end clothing tastes after his several visits to Milan. Derek also was given free shirts from Affliction because he loved their brand and wore their shirts and posted on his social media as he posed in front of the pyramids in Egypt and on the famous bridge in Dubai. He had several thousand followers on Instagram, so Affliction started sending him new arrivals for free. Derek was a savvy guy. He had a Gucci wallet and over a few months purchased several pieces of Gucci clothing and shoes along with Versace sunglasses (he bought me a pair that I cherish) and a Gucci watch. All of it went really well with his F Type 150 Jaguar.

The day after Derek's twenty-eighth birthday in the hospital, after spending another long day there, I left and took his laundry home to wash. One of the things I loved about WakeMed and their rehab program was that patients got dressed every day with normal clothes from home. OT and PT would come by each morning and help him get out of his hospital gown and into real clothes. After Duke, when Derek could start rehab at WakeMed on their neuro rehab unit, I had to go out and buy him stretch pants with elastic waistbands to get on and off easily and go over his diaper. His shirts had to be loose as well both for easy removal and dressing and to accommodate his feeding tube when he couldn't eat. Just a few short months ago, he loved wearing his tight-fitting Gucci shirts and $200.00 jeans with a Gucci belt, his Gucci wallet in his back left pocket and Gucci shoes, his D-Rex hat on while driving his badass Jaguar F-Type. Now he dressed in Hanes stretch pants and baggy T-shirts. This change in his apparel was also painful for me as I couldn't help but feel another piece of Derek was slipping away.

As I empty his plastic bag of clothes from the hospital into the washing machine, soiled from bodily fluids, I feel all the blood rush up to my head and out come the screams, like someone is stabbing me all over my body and dragging a jagged knife down my spine, cutting me in half. I want to claw my face with my sturdy fingers and what little nails I have and bleed out into the washing machine with Derek's soiled clothes and somehow wash away the cancer that was devouring him and relieve the ongoing knife stabbing pain that is killing us.

Chapter 6
Life, Hope, Despair

It is late March 2019. The MRI results look so positive!

Derek has to leave the hospital because the neuro unit and OT/PT have done all they can for him, yet nothing can move on his tired body. Every morning, the OT/PT have come into his hospital room. The hope was to get Derek rehabbed enough so he could go back to the regular rehab floor at WakeMed, where he was at the beginning of this nightmare. One therapist stood on the left side of Derek and the other on the right. They were so kind and gentle with him, asking if anything hurt, letting him know step by step what they would be working on that day. They would get Derek into his clothes, and, if it were a miracle day, they could get Derek in the Hoyer lift and then into his wheelchair. From there, Derek could brush his teeth at the sink. On a double miracle day, after therapy we could then take him outside in his wheelchair for sun and fresh air or to the cafeteria or the gift shop where his favorite candies were. Most OT/PT sessions stopped after both therapists got him from a lying down position in his bed to a sitting position. I would stand behind him because they were training me for when we took Derek home, sharing what we needed to know to keep Derek safe and from falling. When one would let go, Derek would start to tip over; he had no strength to hold his body in any position. I just couldn't believe this was all happening. But it was.

My mind drifts and I remember when we first came onto the neuro unit floor after Duke Hospital. Derek looked in the mirror as he was brushing his teeth. He ran his left hand over the scars on his head. He looked left to right and back and forth for several minutes. He didn't say a word. He just kept staring, the same stare we all had, the *what is happening* stare. I told him his hair would grow back. He looked at me like I was from Mars.

The MRI results are so positive with shrinking tumors, yet things are horribly unbalanced in other ways. His whole body is now completely paralyzed—everything but that left arm. Derek is not able to participate in any sort of rehab. Just trying to reposition him causes glass-like stabbing, jolting pain throughout his thin, tired body. We have hope, so I am busy utilizing my social work skills and advocacy to find out where Derek can go, in hopes another three to four months in a rehab will get some of his body moving again so he can be semi-independent at least.

For some reason, we believe somehow that Derek will end up getting out of that hospital bed and walking to the car and into our home. Talk about blind hope. We are all so dazed and confused, yet we think *somehow* he will get better. Surely being so young, disciplined, an outstanding, compassionate person and a sky soldier will mean he improves. And surely God will hear all the prayers from around the world, and a miraculous healing will happen. Other people have battled cancer and won, and Derek should be no different. It's not like we had fewer prayers than others, less strength than others, because our hearts are all praying and our teeth are sunk into this monster, and we aren't letting go—obviously!

I have found a sympathetic social worker at the VA in the patient rehab program in Durham who is my angel. I go for a visit to see if they can accommodate Derek and his needs. And they can! They have hospital beds that look like a bed from home with nice quilts and fluffed up pillows. There are Hoyer lifts with tracks on the ceiling to safely transfer patients like Derek who can't ambulate to and from the bathroom and bathtub. They have 24/7 nursing care, activity rooms, and an awesome cafeteria with food I know Derek will love. And he can be with other veterans who served their country who now also have bodies that can't move from the war while Derek's mangled body is in the cancer war right here in North Carolina.

I beg and cry, trying to persuade them to accept him for 90 days. Derek does not fit the typical application criteria of this VA program because he is not able to participate in any type of rehab. If they will just agree to accept him, they will give one last try to rehab Derek. It will give us time to get our house retrofitted, time to get a power wheelchair fitted for him and a hospital bed for the living room. We apply for Medicaid so he can qualify for in-home care. This must be a sight to see. Here I am in the Medicaid office at DSS with my husband who is, by the way, the Medicaid Director in North Carolina, going through what every person goes through trying to figure out the application and daunting process of applying for Medicaid. Good grief!

I cannot regurgitate all the frustration of hundreds of hours trying to work with the VA, Derek's health insurance, and other things that the VA should be able to help us with. After all, Derek was in the hospital at Duke for two months and directly across from the VA hospital, a three-minute walk! Derek was out of the Army less than six months before he became sick, and the VA didn't recognize he was a veteran, for Christ's sake. A dear person whom I met in my professional life, Randy, a retired Army Colonel, tries to help. He meets me at the VA's office one day, and we sit for hours, trying to make sense of a system that is so broken. Their departments are in one building, but their computer systems and data do not connect to one another;

I had no idea just how bad it was. My God, people fight for this country, lose lives and limbs, and then they and their families have to go through this bullshit Rubik's Cube process to try to get any assistance with anything at all. You need to have this, match that, copy this, fill out this and take it two doors down, bring it back and wait another two hours only to be told not much; we have to submit it all now and see. See *what*?

The only help we receive is from that angel social worker at the VA. Social workers (99% of them) do not get the credit they deserve. They are not seen as the heroes and frontline workers that many of them are. They face the most daunting challenges, are given cases that people run from, but, you know what, someone has to do it, and social workers just roll up their sleeves, chomp down, and help keep this world glued together. They figure it out and they never give up on people, never. Thank heavens.

Because of that angel social worker, Derek is accepted into the VA program for 90 days, and we can move him there in the next couple weeks. He will receive 24/7 nursing care and therapy services in hopes of rehab until he can come home—finally out of hospital! We plan to use that time to get the house ready and the powered wheelchair fitted for him and purchase an accessible van to get him out and about to doctors' appointments and into the world. Being out of the hospital will be a day to celebrate!!

April 5, 2019: Derek is extremely sleepy. For the past several days, he has had to have bladder scans and a catheter inserted every six hours; it is no longer bothering him when they insert that tube in, no wincing, no groaning, not a flinch. His body is exhausted and he's slipping into a numbing state of nowhere. His muscles that fought so hard to continue to send signals to the brain are either not firing or they are, but his brain is unable to send a signal back that he has to void. Peeing was the last independent function he could do on a good day. This cancer is taking what little is left of his dignity now. That's what this cancer does; it takes oneself, every ounce of it. I am deeply concerned; my stomach starts knotting up. Derek tries to eat some of the hash browns I brought him this morning before we leave the hospital and head to the VA rehab program. I packed up his room the night before and tried my best to explain to him how much happier he will be at the VA. He can hang out with other soldier guys, eat great food, and hopefully get some of his mobility back with OT and PT, and then home we will go. The ambulance is on standby, and we are waiting for the discharge papers so they can transport Derek to the VA. We will finally leave the hospital!

As I tell Derek about the amenities of the VA program, about the game room there, the awesome kitchen with amazing food, Derek's whole body freezes up, his head starts vibrating, then shaking almost robotically as his eyes roll around. I fly out of the room, screaming for doctors to come. Next thing I know, several amazing, loving caring medical people rush into his room, talking loudly.

"Derek, can you hear me. Derek, we are going to help you."

Right before my eyes, Derek's seizure continues for five minutes. There are ten people in the room now. His oxygen drops to 40%.

My God, what is happening?!

Chapter 7
Two Amens

It is April 8, 2019, three days after the seizure, three days after we were happily making plans to transfer Derek to the VA and less than two weeks since the MRI results showed encouraging results. Derek drifts into mostly sleeping. The MRI this time comes back, and it is all so awful so fast. All the tumors are back in his exhausted and fragile body. The doctors at Duke call after they read the results of the MRI and tell Nic and me there is nothing more they can do. There are not any other treatments. Anything further will be more suffering and inhumane.

Nic starts to scream and starts hyperventilating. I grab her and she and I cry. I am sure our screams are heard throughout that rehab floor. Our angel Brenda is with us, and she has tears rolling down her face. I call Dave....

We spent the last two nights at the hospital in his room before moving to the Transitions hospice facility on April 10. The cancer has come back with a vengeance, and there are no other treatments. After MRIs and CT scans, the doctors at both WakeMed and Duke agree, and so do we that Derek cannot withstand any more treatments. The only treatment left would be radiation, and we all knew that regimen would create more suffering with the same outcome, death.

Derek's brain has shut down and has gone into sleep mode, and the lonely left arm that remained so strong has gone to sleep too. In addition to more tumor growth, there are lesions on his liver that were never there before.

I do not have the words to even begin to describe what I feel. I can only describe it as like being stabbed by knives over and over again and then your body lit on fire, the excruciating pain of realizing the finality of those words and the anger and rage that burns through your flesh and into your soul, knowing cancer, these unimaginable tumors, are taking our son, Nic's brother, this beautiful human being who wanted to live life, love life, and make music.

I am so grateful the ambulance staff transporting Derek to hospice allows me to ride in the back with him. Derek opens his eyes only a couple times and closes them again. His brown eyes, once as big as saucers, are now like quarter moons.

He slowly turns his head and says to me, "*I am sorry, Mom, and I love you.*"

I say, "*Derek, you did nothing wrong, my son; you must know that; cancer invaded you. You have been so strong, and I love you so, so much.*"

Shortly after that, we arrive at Transitions. My God, I am taking my son to the place he will die. I begin to panic, and my mind can't stop racing. The ambulance beeps as it backs up, and the stretcher with Derek on it is gently taken out and then brought into the side door of the hospice home. I am so desperate for something to happen to change all of this that I can't breathe. How can I save him from going in there; what have I done; maybe they all are wrong, the doctors, us, maybe we need to keep trying! My mind races a million miles a minute. My God, this can't *really* be happening. Gazing at my beautiful son who is so very sick and fragile, the reality and what brain cancer has done to him comes back fast and furious. Again, deep breath, be strong. He needs you to see him through until his last breath here on earth and as his soul is passed to the heaven to be with God. That is the definition of being a mom. It is never over, we never give up, we will fight to eternity for our babies, and if it means to the passing of our precious child, that no parent should have to bear that cross, then so be it.

On the second day of hospice and before our Chaplain Luis and his wife Linda are leaving for the day, Luis says a prayer that is so beautiful. It is about God's kingdom and where Derek will be going. I do not recall the rest of the words, only to say I feel the feelings of the prayer like a warm blanket wrapping around my body and hugging my heart. After Luis finishes the prayer, he ends it with "Amen."

Then, in a very faint whisper, Derek says, "Amen."

We all are standing there, shocked. Nic slowly bends down and whispers in Derek's ear:

"Derek, what did you just say?"

Again, in a raspy whisper, Derek says, "Amen." Those are the last words Derek speaks.

Over the next few days, friends and family visit, and one of Derek's best friends, his traveling buddy, Nate, drives all the way from Nebraska to say goodbye. He shares with us such fond memories. We listen and crave to hear more. It helps comfort our aching hearts as we wait for Derek to transition to what I pray is a place called heaven. I once believed that there is life after death on this earth, but my faith has been depleted over these past four months. Nate talks about their travels, what a great person Derek is, how Derek could plan a destination and time it out to a tee. Nate calls a couple of Derek's friends, one in Brazil, and puts the phone by Derek's ear so he can hear their goodbyes and their love for him.

It's 4 a.m. on April 17, and I can't sleep. I look at my child in his hospice bed, and I still just cannot believe it. I stare at the several areas on his body that have little ports like little IV lines for administering his medications to keep him comfortable. Then I hear his whispered breathing, and I know it will not be long. I carefully crawl into bed with Derek and cradle him. I smell him and run my hands over his scarred, bald head. I feel the softness of his ears, my trembling hands caressing the shape of his face so I can remember it always. I tell Derek he can let go. I promise there is life after death, and we will see each other again. I tell him how much I love him and thank him for being such a wonderful son. I say how sorry I am for the times I may have disappointed him. I know Derek will not take his last breath with me holding him; he would wait, and he did. I crawl back onto the sleep sofa with Nic and close my tired eyes. I pray Derek will pass, and he does shortly thereafter. I hear the nurse assistant come in to check on him, and she quickly leaves the room.

At 5:48 a.m., Derek lets go. He looks very peaceful. No pain, no moaning, no groaning, no crying, no yelling from excruciating head pain—just peace and quiet.

The nice man from the funeral home comes to take Derek's body. They gently move him to a stretcher. We drape an American flag over his body and follow the man out of the hospice room, B 11, and down the corridor. No matter what area they are working in, the staff at Transitions stand still and bow their heads as we walk by. I play one of Derek's songs he made, "Bring Us Together." Some of the lyrics go like this: "Yep... we are looking for a God to bring us together. We are looking for a God to bring us together. One, two, three. We are looking for a God, looking for, looking for a God to bring us together."

Derek made that song after he traveled to Auschwitz Concentration Camp in Poland back in 2016. He was so disturbed by that visit that he made the song. Such a big heart. As we are making that walk down the long hallway of Transitions, it feels like we are all heading to the electric chair for a crime we did not commit. I think I may vomit.

From the 10th of April until the morning Derek passed away, we had several people come to visit Derek and our family at Transitions, an amazing and beautiful hospice home. Our beloved Chaplain and Derek's battle buddy Luis and wife Linda, who have been there since Derek went into the hospital, had been such a godsend for us and especially for Derek. Luis also served in the Army, and he would call Derek his battle buddy sometimes. Derek's faith in God was present and was seen and felt throughout his four months of living in the hospital. Through his early adulthood, Derek challenged faith, God, the man upstairs. And that is who Derek was, pushing the "whys and the hows," looking for other possible answers, challenging everything. He was his own man, and so many people loved that about him and wished they had the ability he had to just be who he was.

It's inconceivable to even type these words: Derek passed away peacefully on April 17 at 5:48 a.m.

On April 18, 2019, my husband, daughter, and I return from the funeral home. We are all relieved we have a beautiful celebration of Derek's life planned. Words cannot explain just how painful, numbing, and surreal it is to write the obituary for your child and plan his funeral.

I needed a prayer card, something people can take with them to always remember Derek. The picture on the front was easy: him dabbing in Egypt. But I struggled with the message. What would Derek want to say? He is not religious. What would he have wanted to *say* to me, to his family and friends?! I found what I hoped would be something close at least in the underground

Holly Richard

world, the website where many people turn when they or a loved one has been impacted by these WTF tumors. (Readers will learn more about the underground world in Part Three, "Tomorrow.")

Note from Heaven

As I sit in heaven and watch you every day,
I try to let you know with signs I never went away.
I hear you when you're laughing, and watch you as you sleep.
I even place my arms around you to calm you as you weep.
I see you wish the days away, begging to have me home.
So I try to send you signs so you know you are not alone.
Don't feel guilty that you have life that was denied to me.
Heaven is truly beautiful, just you wait and see.
So live your life, laugh again, enjoy yourself, be free.
Then I know with every breath you take
You'll be taking one for me.
Love you from Heaven.

Xoxo Anonymous

YESTERDAY

Chapter 8
Mosh Pit of Grief

I found a website, an underground world of thousands of people and caregivers who were talking, supporting, and pouring out their disbelief and gut-wrenching pain about the enormous and cruel impact of brain cancer. Who knew such a thing existed! We never wanted to be a part of this club, but there we all were. On May 10, 2019, we had an opportunity to reach out to medical professionals in Illinois with questions. This is what I wrote:

My son, 27, was suddenly diagnosed with a primary brain tumor in his left temporal lobe on December 12, 2018. Because of its location and his symptoms of headaches and vomiting, they had to remove most of the tumor on December 14. The initial diagnosis was a poorly differentiated cancerous neoplasm. We were told he would need a few days in the hospital followed by outpatient radiation. A PET scan was done prior to surgery and confirmed there were not any other signs of cancer in his body. My son never left the hospital or ever walked again.

I outlined the timeline for his cancer treatment as follows:

- Surgery was done on 12/14.

1. *Due to the location of tumor, it affected speech and immobilized his entire right side similar to a stroke.*

2. *He began inpatient rehab on 12/26.*

3. *Progress was made with his right side responding well to therapy.*

4. *On 1/4/2019, my son was vomiting, and an MRI was done that showed the tumors were spreading.*

5. *He was transferred to Duke Hospital via ambulance.*

6. *Hydrocephalus was awful and tumors were now located throughout the brain and spinal cord. He was diagnosed with rare hybrid glioblastoma and embryonal tumor.*

7. *A shunt was placed in order to start six weeks of grueling radiation treatments, and then he had another brain surgery to revise the shunt, which held up.*

8. *Temporary feeding tube was done due to nausea and lack of nutrition.*

9. *Treatment was effective at shrinking and killing tumors.*

10. *He was transferred back to WakeMed Hospital neuro unit on 2/28/2019 to get strong enough to start rehab as his left leg now had little strength and his right side was completely immobile.*

11. *Avastin infusions every two weeks were working with few side effects.*

12. *My son was never able to rehab or to walk and was completely dependent on all personal care.*

13. *My son began a quick decline in mental status, sleeping much of the time, and lost use of the only*

moving extremity, his left arm. An MRI at the end of March showed significant improvement with tumors shrinking, and another MRI on April 8 showed new cancer growth. After all the radiation and Avastin, we were losing him.

14. *After three brain surgeries, six weeks of brain and spine radiation, and several infusions of Avastin, he spent four months fighting like the warrior he was, battling what was a rare glioblastoma and embryonal tumor (CNS).*

15. *On April 10, after all treatments to fight this monster cancer were exhausted, the tumors came back, and my precious son passed in hospice on April 17.*

It has been unbearable as those on this site know all too well. I know we all grieve for our losses; parents aren't supposed to write the obituary and plan a service for their child nor are their siblings. Is there anyone that has experienced this type of brain tumor that leaves the brain, travels throughout the CNS, and paralyzes a soldier of nine years so that he cannot leave a hospital bed until hospice? I am desperately looking for answers as to how my healthy son ended up with this monstrosity of cancer. I cannot find other people who experienced this type of tumor that spreads outside of the brain and in cerebral spinal fluid. We were told it is due to cells splitting abnormally, that it was more molecular and very rare and "extremely bad luck." Our docs and medical team have been wonderful, but so much is unknown about this hybrid of a tumor. Please help us understand as bad luck is not an acceptable diagnosis for what took his life.

Sincerely,

Holly, Derek's mom

Holly Richard

Here was their response:

Reply today at 10:59 a.m.:

Hello, Holly. I am so sorry for your loss. Your son's case was not a typical case of glioblastoma. Spread of cancer to the spinal fluid (also called leptomeningeal metastasis) is being reported more frequently in recent years, theoretically because we are getting better control of the primary tumor. There have been no identifiable "causes" of brain cancer, so unfortunately the "extremely bad luck" explanation is the best I can offer. Perhaps other family members who have experienced this devastation will also reach out on this post.

Again, *bad luck*? Are you kidding me? Little babies, five-year-old children, and 28-year-old healthy men and women do not die of bad luck! So I decided I needed to get the geniuses at Duke back around a table with me. I could not save my son—no one could—but I will be damned his life was taken from him due to bad luck. I began calling and emailing the folks at Duke in hopes we could get this meeting set up soon.

* * *

On May 11, 2019, I wrote the following message.

My dear son. I walked the lake again today. For some reason, and I really do not know why, but I felt you there. I know you were there with me. In the quiet moments at the lake, when the breeze hit my face, I could feel you somehow, trying to comfort my hurting heart and lost soul. I cried, and I wrote this poem there.

My Son Is Gone

When I laugh

I want to cry.

When I smile

I want to die.

I cannot breathe.

There is no reprieve

After a loss of a child.

The order of nature

Is so wrong.

Where do I now belong

After a loss of a child?

The child I carried in my womb –

How could he be gone so soon,

Stripped from my arms?

I am overwhelmed with strife.

Cancer cannot take him;

Instead please take my life.

As the sun awakens,

My eyes are open.

The pain is not mistaken;

It feels like I am sinking

Holly Richard

To the bottom of the depthless sea.

As the sun sets,

My heart tries to forget

Until the morning comes,

In its beauty and warmth

That peaks into my window

Quickly turns me ice cold

Knowing today my son is still gone.

© 2019 Holly Richard

May 22, 2019

I have spent the past several days upstairs going through Derek's belongings. The packed and unpacked items that were to be taken to his move to Georgia covered the floor of his music room. Treasures from his many travels, his clothes, and so many of his belongings created so many different thoughts racing through my mind.

I remembered his shoes at home, always in perfect alignment like they were waiting for the drill sergeant to come inspect to make sure they were in perfect formation. As I stared at all of his belongings on the floor, I felt the fear again of my soldier son attacked by cancer. How I wanted to kill it, to kill anything. The beast came out, and the rage made my skin feel on fire. I remembered when I punched the wall until my knuckles bled; then I ran down the hospital hall frantically looking for him. I couldn't find him. My mind raced out of control. He was whisked down for an emergency CT scan, fluid buildup on his brain, hydrocephalus out of control. The pain made him scream my name, and he punched the bed with the only extremity that worked, his left hand. Then he passed out.

The flashbacks stopped. I chose not to keep those shoes, the black sneakers with a red stripe around the sole, his favorite red and black, Atlanta Falcons colors. The last memory of those shoes in that hospital room was not where my heart wanted to go, so I put them in the black donation bag. You may wonder why I would keep that radiation mask, the one I referenced earlier, that looked like something out of a Stephen King thriller, that mask I so dreaded seeing pass by me every day for six long weeks, knowing my son would be strapped into that thing. You see, when they made the mask, they molded it to Derek's face; it was custom made. I sat there with the mask for a while and hugged the mask over and over again. I felt his ears and nose were right where they should be, it was the outline of Derek's beautifully shaped features. I held it just like I had when I cradled him at hospice and when curled up in his hospital bed, feeling all of his features so I would never forget. Just like I did when he was little when he fought sleepy time. I would rock him for hours as he nestled his little face against my neck and I caressed his head, cheeks, his ears and then patted his back.

I moved on to his T-shirts with so many funny expressions, and I had a brief chuckle. These T-shirts were so Derek and showed his enormous sense of humor. The sayings on his shirts— everything from "I Could Cuddle You So Hard" to "Stay Calm and Jump" to "Pickle Rick" and "Rick and Morty." I smelled them and squeezed the cloth as hard as I could to get every scent of his skin that breathed into that fabric. I wished I could bottle it and spray it everywhere and make candles with the smell of Derek.

I looked at his sunglasses, Oakley's, of course, and put them on. What did this child see through these glasses; where had he walked with those shoes? Traveler that he was, Derek went so many places, some all by himself. I don't read books; my attention span is that of a gnat, yet I bought one a couple weeks ago having no idea that some of Julie's story in the book, as different as her life's journey was, revealed that she and Derek were fighting their own cancer beast. Their travels around the world gave them their warrior armor and their willingness to face it head on. Also, with a sense of living so much, so fast and being so young, she conveyed a sense of being okay if life had to end here on earth.

Julie Lip Williams was diagnosed out of nowhere with stage IV colon cancer in her thirties. Like Derek, the diagnosis of death. The chance of Julie getting such a diagnosis and at such an early age was like .000000000000000000000000000008%. (That may be too many zeros, but you get the picture.) She was a traveler too, and she explained the absolute adrenaline, confidence, the autonomy, the curiosity, and the accomplishment of feeling "I can do anything" on her travels.

I knew Derek experienced the same adrenaline high. He went to 25 countries by the age of 25, and he did that in less than three years. This child did not drive over the speed limit for fear, yes, fear, of being pulled over by a police officer for speeding. I am serious, and my husband can back me, and, of course, I have driven with Derek many times and it was true. Yet when it came to travel, he would plan his trips as carefully and meticulously as Picasso would stroke colors and bring shapes to life. Travel was Derek's art, and his music he made from these travels were his vessels to share with the world what it was like. Julie's journeys and Derek's travels had given them the strength and confidence to look down cancer's barrel and say, "Bring it on!"

My mind then traveled to me dragging black trash bags of clothes to the local laundromat at age 17. I don't know why, but there I was back in South Florida in 1979. Not many teenagers at 17 were on their own, 1,200 miles from home, dragging 50 pounds of jeans to a laundromat with a friend named Scam, who, by the way, wore a boa constrictor (Clyde) around his neck everywhere he went. That is a true story. Clyde lived with us too, and he didn't have a cage so to speak. Clyde would often hang from the curtain rod, sometimes the chandelier. Clyde would sleep at night in a pillowcase in Scam's top dresser drawer. Crazy, but what is even crazier was Natasha, our pet Tarantula. She lived in a small aquarium with a screened lid, and we would often take her out to hold her. I was fascinated by her. Holding her in my hand, she would sit and let me pet her on her back end, her opisthosoma (I confess, I had to look that up). All the time I knew that underneath her, directly touching my hand were her fangs that could bite me at any time! My then boyfriend, Ron, who later became my husband and father of our children, bought her when she was a baby. The first time I held her, she hauled ass up my arm and sat on my neck. I have a Polaroid picture of that. I was 15 years old at the time. I was so afraid yet wildly entertained and had the dangerous curiosity of wondering if she would bite my throat with her tarantula fangs!

We had Natasha for 13 years. When Nicole was born, we put Natasha's aquarium out in the shed. I was a mom then; my parental instincts were kicking in. Who would have a pet tarantula in their home with a baby in the house? Now I scratch my head and think, who would ever have a snake or a tarantula in their home period! Natasha was so very tame and never bit anyone, and, believe me, we had some parties where she was held by a lot of people, and we had to go looking through the house to find her the next day! Still, I took no chances, and the shed was a good place for Natasha to live out her remaining years.

While teenagers were cramming for tests, getting ready for proms, searching for colleges, eating dinner around the table with family, I was far away from family, living with my boyfriend whom I later married and had two precious children with: Nicole and Derek. Yep, there I was on my own. I quit high school in my junior year, although I immediately took the GED and passed it. I needed to get to work. My first job was picking up dog poop outside the kennel for a veterinarian. I wanted to be a veterinarian when I was a small child who never really got to be a child. I quickly moved on from picking up dog doodoo to becoming a sandwich artist, making subs, good ones at that. I worked split shifts and each day I had a three-hour break. Since I didn't have a car or a driver's license, I was stuck there during my break. Boredom was never my friend, so I would voluntarily clean the place.

Nothing was ever easy for me growing up, so I expected everything in my life to be hard. That was my norm, especially after my mother and father divorced when I was 11 years old. Every day felt like a sink or swim marathon. But motherhood was what kept me alive throughout various lows in my life. I was far from a perfect mom in the beginning, and I had my share of *I wish I did that instead of that* and a few, *what was I thinking* moments! I was young but eventually started to figure out how to be not just mom, but a good mom. I lived for and through my children. I read books and articles on all the things the psychologists and pediatricians said to do and not to do. I did my best to teach them to always practice the Golden Rule, and I taught about consequences of the choices they made. I eventually went to college at age 36 after having two active children who played multiple sports while I was working full time. It took me seven *long* years to get my bachelor's degree, but I knew I needed that education to get me through the door of the nonprofit world of helping people. I was fortunate I was able to take out loans so I could go to college. So many people cannot afford to go; it just isn't fair. I think our country should at least make community colleges free for everyone and paid for in well-thought-out strategies. It can be done, people!

I remember when Nicole was about eight years old, she would not stop running around the pool, and I knew it was just a matter of time before she wiped out and skinned her knees. When she would not listen to my shouts to stop running, I gave her a smack on the butt. She looked up at me with those big brown eyes, the same beautiful eyes that Derek had, and her facial expressions told me there had to be a better way. I never spanked her again. Derek never had a spanking in his life. Was he spoiled—yes! Even when he was little, he would get so frustrated and would throw his hot wheel cars through windows when they fell off the track. No spanking, but the absence of his hot wheel cars for a couple days made him think twice about it, and eventually he stopped. My children always knew at the end of the day how I felt about them. I would say, "I love you; I am there for you and to protect you. I love you no matter what!" They understood that I would never, ever abandon them.

Brain cancer challenged us all to the core. My battle scars of childhood did not give me the strength, but they did give me the pain to survive. Unconditional love of a mother for a child, that bond that cannot be broken, helped me to encourage, love, and protect my son, to learn about this cancer, become a teammate with the medical staff and nurses, know the medicine and administration of it as well as they did. I love my children, and cancer took my son, and an eating disorder was wreaking havoc on my precious daughter. I was in a dark place writing this, experiencing the ultimate fear of being childless. How could this be happening? All I ever wanted to be was a mother and grandmother. I felt scared to death.

Chapter 9
Another Way Around

After Derek's first brain surgery to remove what was the one and only primary tumor at that time, his brain had to figure out how to reroute, to discover another way to find words from different places, and to reroute again to send thinking instructions via a whole different path to talk, to put sentences together that weren't word salad, to try and move his right leg, arm, to move anything on his body. After Derek died, I found myself having to search for a way around the massive pothole in my heart from losing my child so I could open my eyes, get out of bed, and navigate new ways around my upside-down life. I wondered how to reroute this pain to move forward. Like Derek's arms and legs, my pain remained in place, no movement; it couldn't redirect to anywhere either.

More images of Derek went through my mind: Derek from the top of the Alps, riding camels in Egypt, exploring the pyramids, doing the Dab (a move that musicians and some athletes do when performing for a crowd or conquering their opponent), at the Great Wall of China, chasing rainbows in Sparta, and fish sucking his toes in a spa in Florence with precious girlfriend Alice. These fleeting pictures would bring a short-lived smile, and then cancer would beat me over the head again and jerk me back to reality.

Nic, too, had been rerouting, trying to find another way around so much pain from having to watch her only sibling go through such hell. Then she had to be on guard 24/7 with her eating disorder (ED). She had to wake up every morning and creep through the ED tunnel, thinking about ED all day, wondering when it might ambush her like the *Predator* movie, invisible and then not.

In my search for more and more answers I needed about the monster cancer, I was able to get a meeting at Duke on May 23, 2019, with some pretty amazing medical professionals. That word underrated them because they were geniuses, the heroes who fought cancer every minute of every day. My guardian angel, Brenda Wilcox, the transitional care navigator for oncology for both WakeMed and Duke, who had been with us since Derek got off the ambulance at WakeMed prior to his first surgery, helped set up the meeting. It took weeks, but, hell, I would have waited until hell froze over.

The meeting started promptly at 9:30 that morning. Dr. Desjardins, associate professor of neurology at Duke, who orchestrated and planned the strategy and attack of these tumors, was there. She was barely five feet in height but so much taller in her presence. It felt she could bolt through the ceiling like *Alice in Wonderland*. That is how her presence appeared in my eyes.

Dr. Leslie Thomas, the Duke hospitalist, could not be there. She and I spent each day from January 4 through February 28 attached at the hip—almost—so much so that there were days when I briefed her on the status of Derek when she rotated off every other weekend. She was another brilliant doctor with an amazing bedside manner. She had no problem kneeling down to look at me when I was so weary I could not lift my head enough to make eye contact. On countless occasions, she curled up on the sofa bed next to me in Derek's hospital room to talk and listen and throw out ideas on the course of treatment and care for Derek. She was the eyes and ears of the behind-the-scenes doctors. To distract my overheated mind, she also shared stories about her standing in the driveway at her apartment complex at 2:00 a.m. because the fire alarm went off. She was real, she was special, and Derek trusted her, and so I did too.

In one of our many conversations while Derek was at Duke, she told me that I had earned my minor degree in medicine. How I wish I never had to take those courses, but there was nothing I would not do for my son. The minor degree consisted of the following courses: hands-on work, personal care, counseling, overseeing shift changes, communication, communication, communication, pain management, food, nutrition, and overall personal and emotional care strategies along with becoming aware of a whole host of personnel, a small army of them.

This took into account not just neurology, oncology, hospitalist docs, surgeons, and the resident doctors but also the nurses, nurse assistants, and the "lift team," who would swoop in when needed to turn Derek every two hours. (He never got a bed sore in four months!). It also included X-ray personnel, blood draw technicians, technicians who had to stick all those suction cups on Derek's head to monitor for seizures and had to come back the next day to take them off. (As they peeled those adhesive suction cups off of his bald and scarred head, Derek would yell and say, "Knock it off. What the fuck did I ever do to you?!") Add to the list housekeeping and kitchen staff and Radiation Oncologist Dr. John Kirkpatrick, who was also brilliant and had a heart bigger than his chest could hold. He couldn't be there for the meeting. Neither could Neurosurgeon Dr. Allan Friedman. I am not sure what kind of feeling I would have had if God walked into my room, but Dr. Friedman had that presence. After all, his installation of Derek's shunt, followed by a revision to replace and install a low-pressure valve shunt to handle all the dead WTF tumors, was remarkable as was his radiology department and their army of techs and nurses.

Then there were the transport personnel, the people who took Derek everywhere via his bed when he left the hospital room to travel the many tunnels in the hospital when he needed CT scans, MRIs, and radiation every morning at the cancer center. Derek was not able to move or sit up and was totally dependent on transport to drive his bed to and from these tests. There were also the OT, PT, and speech therapists, the dietician, acute pain consultants, the palliative care team with nurse practitioners, LCSWs, the chaplain, and the cancer family therapist. This was only the Duke Army and did not include any of the minor degrees I earned at WakeMed.

You get the idea: brain cancer was hideous. The brain is so complex, and in just one day a person with brain cancer can go from feeling awesome to awful to periods of feeling better to feeling awful to critical condition, back to stable, back to full-blown tumors, to hospice. It was a roller coaster from hell that no one should ever be on, especially a 28-year-old, my precious son, a rare and beautiful person who had this rare and relentless brain cancer.

Dave, Nic and I sat at the small table with Dr. Desjardins and Brenda while Dr. Desjardins led discussions of the assumptions, opinions, and new findings about this tumor that belonged to Derek. One of the reasons I could not find anyone on this planet that had a tumor that behaved the same way is that, until 2016, the medical geniuses could not even define what it was. It now has a name, the glioblastoma with IDH (Isocitrate dehydrogenase) mutation, which I think is the IDH wildtype (that was a real type). I may not have this description of the tumors accurate, so do not hold it against me, please. I left that whole WTF type of tumor and what it was made of to others. Like I said, I'm not getting into specifics on something so sci-fi and unimaginable. So we moved on to the heart of the meeting: Derek.

I asked, if it really multiplied so fast, was it really cells dividing in which the DNA wasn't right, so the cells turned to abnormal cells? The answer was "yes" to these questions. Next thing we knew, Dr. Desjardins left the room and returned with *the* Dr. Henry Friedman. Yes, neuro oncologist for Ted Kennedy and other well-known people whom he had treated who also had the dreaded cancer X on their backs. And there we were, with wonderful people in the room who fought this beast with Derek sitting with me, Dave, and Nic. Our meeting was about what comes next; how could Derek's life and death make a difference in education, awareness, research? I knew Derek was smiling somewhere, knowing his family was going to keep on keeping on until we made the world better so others will not have to suffer or can be pre-screened as children when it comes to brain tumors. May the world be saved from this torturous hell that Derek and our family had to endure.

* * *

My time alone with Dave was so needed. As we lay together that morning before getting ready to head back home, we were able to have our bodies embraced with the pure love of each other. As I rested my head on his chest, I ran my fingers through his chest hair and down his scars from three heart surgeries. I was more in love with him than ever. And he hugged me like it was the last time he would see me. He had been so strong for me and Nic. He had very little emotional support, and he was grateful for the support from our chaplain, our protector who waited quietly at the hospitals and then showed up when we needed him most. Dave had been a pillar of strength. He had a huge job, and I really do not know how he had been able to work and be present for Derek, Nic, and me over the past four months. He hadn't sought out therapists and support groups as I had frantically been doing. They were my oxygen tanks, and I could not have breathed otherwise. I was afraid of where my mind would go if I didn't seek that kind of assistance. I needed to be strong for Nic. I was so scared I would become a mother without children. My childhood fueled my intense desire to live with and through my children. Nic had been fighting her battle with ED, and I could somehow help her at times when I could see it in her; we could combat that terrorist. Unlike cancer, the predator and coward.

Our hugs and closeness soothed our aching souls as we melted into each other. The chances of us finding each other to love and to hold in this big world were less than winning the lottery. I thank God Dave survived his one massive heart attack at age 32 followed by two more heart attacks before the age of 34. Hearts and brains are so fragile and complicated.

* * *

May 30, 2019: Recurring Hope

Sometimes I forgot just how exhausting those four months had been for us. I also saw the exhaustion and sadness with the treatment team of the many who cared for Derek after he passed away. Nic and I went to Duke that morning to meet with Dr. Kirkpatrick, the radiology oncologist who could not be there at our first meeting. He had spent every day with Derek and me for six weeks, shooting the hell out of those tumors, the gremlins, the little cowards. He had cried with us and fought fiercely with Derek's ongoing battle with brain tumors, and thank God there were people like these doctors, committed to doing this day after day. Nic and I thanked the good doctor and headed to the Eighth

West floor at Duke. We hugged our nurses and doctors who had cared for Derek. He left such a mark on everyone's heart. We walked by his room, B12, where I spent every day from January 4 through February 28. I looked out the window where I had sobbed every day as I listened to the caregivers trying to refresh and change Derek and heard his cries from the pain that were at times excruciating, where every nerve in his body must have felt like glass cutting or like being electrocuted. The smallest move of his body could send him screaming. Dilaudid would save the moment, and sometimes they had to also administer Ativan straight into the vein. Then we watched his face until the drugs numbed the pain so Derek could have a reprieve.

After meeting with Dr. Kirkpatrick at Duke, Nic and I went to WakeMed, where Derek spent two and a half months. We went to floor 2C first and hugged the OT and PT therapists, Emily and Christie. We gave them a prayer card from Derek's funeral. They worked incredibly hard and gave Derek and us so much hope when Derek was there the first time. After Derek's first brain surgery, he was recovering; he stood up and held onto the parallel bars. With their expertise, Derek was able to get out of that hospital bed and out of the wheelchair; he didn't need a Hoyer lift to do so, and he was rehabbing like he was dabbing. Look at me now!

Then we went up to neuro on the sixth floor. There was Nurse Chris, who was from Italy, and Carrie, the nurse assistant, who would come and visit Derek even when she was assigned to a different floor. She called him the most appreciative patient she ever had. We shared a few tears and hugged and thanked them. I do not know if other families return to these hospital floors to visit these heroes who were out of the spotlight. What they do is so profound and unbelievable. They took such good care of Derek, they loved him fiercely too, and they were forever changed by Derek. Nurse Chris called Derek's a "strong story" that punched him sometimes as he remembered. We didn't get to see our awesome Nurse Connie, who was there almost every day with us too. Derek had many followers on this journey, not just from Instagram and Facebook and followers around the world, but also doctors, nurses, assistants, therapists. The list was long.

Nic and I walked by what was once Derek's room, 6B36, and the open wounds of our hearts started pouring out pain from missing him, for all he went through, all we went through as we also remembered the tender moments and even a few funny stories that would forever linger in our minds. Because Derek ended up with aphasia after the first brain surgery and then more surgeries that followed, his communication and cognitive and intellectual ability changed drastically. He was not the same Derek, yet he was. There were times where Dave, Nic, and I would have to get our charades skills out to guess what he was saying. There were times where it deflated Derek's whole being, and other times where he would smile and give a thumbs up when we guessed what he was saying or asking, and we would all laugh together. Usually he was asking for something to eat, and "USA" was the word he used to describe food.

Nic and I could not stare long into the room as there was another lady sitting in that same windowsill with her loved one in the bed that Derek lived in most of every day as of just a few weeks ago. We walked on and stopped, hugged, and cried. Our memories of this horrible and painful time and the brain cancer that attacked every cell in his body like piranha, waiting for each cell to divide and then kill it, also reminded us of the pure love for Derek and his caregivers and how much we all tried with everything we had to save him somehow.

On June 20, 2019, I worked some more on cleaning out Derek's room. It was awful and made the actuality all the more real; he was gone from my sight. It reminded me of the feeling when you lose sight of your small child in a store and your heart beats so hard you think you'll pass out. Your mind goes immediately to an abductor, a child molester taking your child. So many haunting scenarios flood your mind until you become hysterical. That is what it felt like for me. The grieving process intensifies every time I open my eyes in the morning and realize my beloved child is gone from my sight. A parent just cannot grasp that concept—sort of like the bad luck theory. I hate cancer!

* * *

Seeing red, white, and blue used to send wave after wave of pride through me until I felt I would burst. My soldier son served this country. Now, on the 4th of July, seeing the colors of America made me so sad, angry, and empty. Instead of having a cookout in the backyard, we visited the cemetery, putting patriotic flowers and flags on Derek's grave. I found myself still in shock all over again and could not fathom that he was really gone from our lives. I realized I was in identity crisis mode. I was Derek and Nicole's mom, but now half of me was gone. I did not know who I was anymore. What should I do now? Where did I belong? Everything that once mattered no longer seemed important. I felt more anger as my wounds remained exposed from this horrible nightmare, the cancerous dungeon that I'd landed in. Why Derek? How? It just can't be so.

Yet it was. Once again my heart was racing to find another way around the pain, a place where it could hide from the piercing grieving knives, but there was nowhere to hide. I was surrounded by this darkness, this hell where chains were hung on me that I dragged everywhere I went. I felt like a leper; people avoided me, wondering what to say to me, the grieving mother.

The silence was deafening sometimes. People who I thought would be there through thick and thin quietly stepped back into their world, avoiding mine. After all, what could you say to a mother who had a front-row seat to her son's death as she watched helplessly while he was being swallowed by these tumors for 126 days until his last breath? We sat by his bedside, helplessly trying to find the magic cocktail of medicine, treatments, something, but nothing could save my Derek. I watched and I watched and I watched day after day. What could anyone say to a parent who went through this and who continued to go through this? How does anyone go through this and come back to life? Was this life now? I felt numb. I was afraid of the quiet anger that continued to bubble. That anger that despises parents with grown sons who were married as they enjoyed their grandchildren, parents who could see their beautiful son's eyes in a little remake of him. I would never see that nor feel those little arms wrap around my neck as Derek's once did when I rocked him to sleep as he fought the sleepy nighttime, refusing to give up on the day, getting every second he could before sleep crept in. I felt so envious of people who had those little feet running in the house, the giggles and laughter, the magic of Santa and the Easter bunny. This misplaced awful anger and grief! I could not stop the madness in my head.

Chapter 10
The Wall

I saw it ever so closely, that wall that I brought with me and let float alongside me at times since Derek passed away. It was back, and it made me shake so much to even flip an eye up to it, that monstrous feeling of someone no longer present, gone from this life, my son, just gone. Again and again, I said it in my mind. My shoulders leaned inward, and somehow I thought I could annihilate that wall, knowing the pain crushing every bone in my body was welcomed because it could never compare to the million pieces of my glass heart, shattered inside me, cutting my ligaments and joints right down to my bones and into my soul.

I was at home on a Monday evening, July 8, at 6:30. Derek would have been downstairs talking about the day and the plan for dinner. I didn't think I could stay in this home anymore, the place where Derek was ever so present. The upstairs was all his. His smell lingered in the atmosphere, and I could still envision him walking through the rooms. Sometimes I looked upstairs and felt the same way as I did about the wall. *He can't be gone; he just can't.*

On July 17, 2019, GBM Awareness Day, I woke at 3 a.m.; it had been three months since Derek passed. What did that mean; how could he be gone? Those questions played over and over in my head like old records that would skip when the album was scratched. The skipping and popping sound never stops unless you pick the arm up off the record player. I had to pick myself up to get out of bed that morning. I needed to go to Wilmington for work and to see the staff and celebrate their amazing dedication. I didn't fall back to sleep. Instead, I let the record player keep skipping, and I found this letter I sent to Derek.

October 4, 2015

Hello my dear son,

I hope you are doing well. I miss you so much, but I am so proud of you and that you are seeing the world and serving this great country!! I know your days must be really hard at times, dealing with so much in the military that we civilians will never truly know the depths of. But I know what a good man you are, and you have to be so strong, yet you have that big heart that makes you so uniquely special, and my son, of course.

We are so looking forward to you coming for Christmas. I will be sure to have time off so we can all be together. I went ahead and paid for your registration for your motorcycle renewal, but since it was not inspected, they would not renew it. But the letter said they will hold the credit on your account, and once you get it inspected, you can just go to the DMV and get your renewal stickers. I saved the letter so you will have that. The bike is in storage in a crate still, so I assume you can get it out of the crate and then store it back there if you take it for a spin over the holiday. We are going to be looking for a home and hopefully buy one and move in by January/February. Then we can store the bike there if we have a garage.

Things are busy here as usual. Dave's job as the new Medicaid director for the state has kept him busy, but he is doing really well. Nic is working hard and traveling; she is on her way to

Chicago today. Dylan is good and with Bekah, they both have been traveling between work and fun, so we do not see them much.

My job is going well and busier than ever. We have our golf tournament coming up on the 19ᵗʰ. I was invited by my college at Western Carolina University to be a part of their Leadership Summit, so I spent two days there and came back yesterday. It was a really great experience and an honor to work along the side of some really successful alumni and the chancellor of the college himself. It was too funny because Dr. Gillespie (you played soccer with his son Aaron) was there as well.

I think of you every day and cannot wait to see you!! We are saving $ so we can visit you in Italy in May or June of next year!

All my love to you, son,

Mom xo

How could he be gone; how did this all happen? The record played over and over in my head. Just when I thought I could not hold on by my nails any longer, feeling like I would drop from the cliff and splatter my guts like a water balloon, I read a beautiful prayer that a mom on the American Brain Tumor Association (ABTA) website sent for all of us who suffered through the war of watching our loved ones get devoured by these WTF tumors, these predators and cowards. It eased the wound for a bit.

I joined a Facebook (FB) page called Helping Parents Heal. We all had lost such precious children, and it was absolutely daunting to read the posts at times. Scroll after scroll after scroll of children, beautiful faces full of life, gone. There was a lot of talk about "mediums" on this FB site, so Nic and I made our way to Charlotte to see a medium that one of my board members swore by. Neither Nic nor I had ever been to one. We agreed we would not tell her anything about who we lost. We went in guarded and skeptical yet hoping to hear something that would prove us wrong. Could we really connect with Derek in the afterlife? We missed him so much that we were willing to try.

I can tell you I left there a bit less skeptical than when I walked into her little home that sat across from the railroad tracks. She lived in a cute little country town where everyone looked after everyone. The medium described in great detail the pain Derek experienced in his face, his paralysis, his intense spirit, and that my cousin Cheryl was there with us in spirit. Cheryl was the first cousin to pass away in Aunt Nancy's family over 25 years ago. Cheryl was like an older sister to me, and she was my maid of honor at my first wedding when I married my children's father. There were other names and events that she talked about that were not anywhere on social media.

I was so worn out; I was on overload. I needed to stop thinking and talking and breathing death and dying. But how?

As much as I loved my work at the Tammy Lynn Center and the amazing, caring, loving staff and the people and families we served, I was beyond exhausted. Grief had become my full-time job. It was the first time I had ever stepped down from a job or anything else that I loved so dearly. I never did that. But I knew I had to take care of myself and be there for Nic as much as I could. I also understood that the center needed and deserved a leader that could give 110% each and every day, and I had to give my 110% to grief. I was on extreme overload.

I could not believe it had been over four months since I wrote. On December 8, 2019, I penned this letter to Derek:

My dear Derek,

Tonight at 7 p.m., I hope you saw the world light up as the people who are left behind lit their candles to show their immense love, sadness, and celebration of those who have passed. There were many lighting a candle for you as you are so loved and touched so many lives.

I could not go to the Compassionate Friends' candlelight service tonight because it would mean that you are truly gone. I am not able to comprehend, understand, accept, whatever it is called. I cannot believe that you have passed on and have gone to heaven. I watched in awe as you were born and I heard you, felt you, outside of my womb for the first time. It was something indescribable, and I hope and pray that same feeling is what happens when we leave this earth and that you felt the same unmeasurable elation on April 17th as we watched you leave this earth as I did the day you and Nicole were born into this world and became my world.

My heart is still in a million pieces. It will be something I will be gluing back, piece by piece, each day for as long as this life journey lasts. It will never be the same heart nor could it. A mother gives birth to a child and then watches that same child take their last breath. How could my heart ever be the same? I know you want me to move forward, and I know how much you love me and want me to not be sad and cry. I know all of that in my head, but a mother's unconditional and undying love for a child cannot come to terms with the fact that her child is gone. I am not sure we ever will.

As I light my candle tonight for you, my son, I do so with such pride for the wonderful young man you are, how fun and

Holly Richard

loving you are, the millions of smiles and hugs you gave to me over 28 years, how brave, strong, and compassionate you are, how intense, sensitive, and unique you are, and how forever grateful I am that God picked me to be your mom.

All my love always & forever,

Mom

On December 24, 2019, I penned another letter.

My dear son, I wrote this poem for you for our Christmas day prayer.

As We Say Your Name

As we say your name,

We shall always remember the wonderful man you are.

As we say name your name,

We honor and thank you for the service to our country.

We are the home of the free

Because of the brave.

You, son, are the bravest of all.

As we say your name,

We remember you for the strong and caring person you are,

For being such a loving son, brother, and friend.

In the coming of Christmas,

We say your name aloud

As you are forever in our hearts and our family.

We say your name at the dinner table

So we will always remember you and carry you

With us until we meet again in heaven.

Derek Ray, loving son, brother, friend,

As we say your name, we remember.

© 2019 Holly Richard

* * *

It's December 29, 2019, and somehow we made it through the Christmas week. It was a blur at times. At other times, I just feel so sad, and then I'm okay and then not. That is how life is once you lose a child. That part of your being has been removed, carved out, like peeling off the tough skin of a vegetable, the protective outer shell, which, once removed, your gaping wound is exposed. I have to learn how to regrow that hard outer skin again. It won't ever be the same texture, nor will it be as strong and resilient. It is

Holly Richard

a different skin, one that is crafted specifically for those who lost a part of their being, their soul, their heart, their existence.

This week, I came across a letter I wrote to Derek the first year he was stationed in Italy.

November 1, 2015

Dear Derek,

I hope all is going well. I think it is so neat that you can DJ and do something fun away from the day-to-day military life. I know your job isn't what you had hoped for there, but seeing the world sure has been a fantastic opportunity for you and at such an early age. I think about that all the time, and I will never in my lifetime see all that you have nor will most of the family on both sides!! I thought this puzzle was really cool since you were there where this picture was taken.

We are so excited you will be home for Christmas! Nic and I have all the time off while you are here, and Dave should have a lot too. We have been house shopping a lot and found the perfect home yesterday (we looked at it a couple times) and made an offer. Well, the same day so did someone else, so now we are waiting to hear back!! It is a really beautiful home. We shall see. I will keep you posted. If we are fortunate to get the home; we would be moved in by the time you get here, which means you can then store your bike in the garage. The home is about five minutes from the apartment complex we used to live in when I first moved to Raleigh – great location!

Dave is off to Washington, DC, for a Medicaid directors meeting with other directors from the USA. He is very excited you are coming home too; maybe the weather will allow for a golf day to Knights Play for all of us. Goodnights Comedy Club is also a fun night if you haven't been. Well, going to get some work done before Monday comes. I love you with all my heart; I am so proud of the man you have become, and always keep your chin up and eyes to the sky.

All my love,

Mom

How I wished to God I could rewind back to that time, that year, that very moment. How much more I would have told him—if only I had known.

* * *

On the last day of 2019, I wrote again to Derek.

Dear Derek,

I am dreading going into 2020 as it will be the first year since 1991 where you have not lived on this earth with us. I just cannot fathom this cruel reality. How can this truly be?

Your cell number is no longer in service. I cannot fathom it. When I couldn't reach your voicemail, trying to swallow was like forcing down a jagged rock that tears you from the inside out. How can it be? How I wish I could call you, just one more time, and hear your voice. When the cell service disconnection happened, I panicked. I never want to forget that gentle, strong voice.

Holly Richard

I read an article recently where a neurologist was referring to certain types of brain tumors comparing them to vampires, feeding on brain activity.

* * *

We were into the first day of 2020, and who really cared? The world, once on its axis, was tilted like a pinball machine. Once you jerk the machine around too much, the sounds go silent. (I know this because I spent my early teenage years living above a pool hall and participated in many pinball competitions and billiards for spending money.) Once the lights shut down, the pinball machine becomes dark, and that little shiny pinball rolls down the middle into an empty hole. You cannot use the flippers to keep the ball in play anymore. Death had come, tumors had taken my son, the world had lost all its vibrant colors and shapes, and it was all pale and full of air, space, empty, lifeless, shapeless, weightless.

After the finality, the obituary, funeral, and burial, I found myself in the middle of nowhere. Mind numbing, heart shattering—grieving the loss of a child was all of that wrapped up in one atomic bomb, obliterating every molecule of my being. There I stood in the middle of nowhere, where I tried to piece back together my body, my burnt flesh, arms, legs, fingers, heart pieces and lungs, cramming eyeballs back into my sockets. I could not hear anything, feel anything; it was unfathomable. The mind and heart could not process such an explosion of grief, that out of order death. It was impossible.

* * *

This poem came from my heart on January 4, 2020.

A Mother Is Given a Son in 1991

The calendar has flipped to 2020

And the first you have not lived

Since you were born in 91.

I knew as soon as I looked at you

That I was the chosen one.

I would be your mom

Who fought for years to have you.

Little did I know

That I would have to fight

To keep you.

That first cry was the most joyous sound;

How truly happy we'll be.

A mother was given a son

In 1991.

A son whom I watched

Holly Richard

As a baby trying to crawl.

When crawling was not fast enough,

Up and running he had become.

Little did I know

You came into this world with such resilience.

You were living in the moment

Ever since I gave you birth.

By two you were swinging a club

Like the Tiger Woods we watched.

By three you were catching the football

Like a little NFL receiver.

By the time you were five,

You met your love of soccer,

A sport that kept you going at the speed of light,

And the adrenaline you couldn't get enough of.

Then came the electronics,

And a gamer you became,

Even entering contests and beating adults.

You were a gamer of the night,

And everyone wanted you on the team.

And then came the blow

When mom and dad divorced.

It was a wound that never healed,

And into music you would find your solace,

For there you were the ruler,

The artist, the master of one,

To make any kind of music

And nurturing it like a son.

The music kept you going,

And then there came the day

When you felt the need to serve.

How proud was I to see you

Graduate basic training

In Oklahoma of all places.

Then to see you graduate from Ft. Gordon,

The communications man,

And then on to get your 82nd airborne wings at Ft. Benning

That I had the honor to pin on.

And to Ft. Bragg you would spend

Six years proudly served

Holly Richard

Graduate from warrior leadership

And a host of medals.

Having you home on weekends when you could

Was amazing and yet

Taken for granted.

Little did I know then

I would lose my son I birthed in 1991.

Reluctantly I bought you that sweet, red motorcycle.

You rode it like an Avenger.

Then to Italy you went,

And there your music raged

By making others happy

To hear what you have made,

And to travel to 25 countries

By the time you turned 25.

I just can't help but wonder,

Who else was by your side?

Through your eyes

I got to travel in time with you

To several wonders of the world.

My traveling man, soldier son,

What a fine young man you have become!

And then you returned home.

How happy we all were

And to start your next chapter,

Attending college with your GI bill

So you could further your love for music.

And then there in the shadows,

We were ambushed by this monster.

The brain tumor invaded your body

And began devouring all it could.

Yet you fought back

Like the warrior you were

And face to face took it on full force

and like a race it became.

You fought it hard without relief,

And it didn't take you down.

Instead, you went down swinging;

You took the beast to its grave.

© Holly Richard 2019

Written to my beautiful son Derek, from mom.

Chapter 11
We Who Grieve Are Not Strong

A friend (another widowed mom who lost a son way too soon) sent me this on January 19, 2020, and it is so spot on. I was given permission to include it in this book.

We Who Grieve Aren't Strong; We're Trying to Survive

We recently lost a dear family member to a lifelong illness at just twenty-three years old. As his devastated father and I were exchanging dozens of texts during those first days following his death: details about the memorial service and speakers who would offer reflections and the minutia of the printing of the program—he interrupted the seeming ordinary of the conversation with a sobering two-word declaration.

This blows.

And then he returned to the logistics of the funeral.

That's it. That's the reality of this kind of loss. Despite what we may want to be true about grief, there really are no silver lining life lessons or detached moments of perspective that shield your heart from the scattering shrapnel of grief.

It's just horrible.

It's just a nightmare.

It just blows.

After you lose someone you love, people often tell you they admire your strength. They say it with great affection and with the sweetest of intentions. They say it because they genuinely believe it to be true.

They're also always wrong.

The death of a person you shared your life with immediately places you in a very specific community: you become a *survivor*. This isn't an accolade you earn or a title you work for; it's simply your status now. Someone dear to you has left and you are still here—just trying to survive the horrible event of their departure.

A couple of months after my father died, my mother relayed a conversation she had while running into a distant relative in the grocery store. After an awkward exchange of small talk that eventually stumbled into the topic of the dead elephant in the room, the person complimented my mother:

"I admire you." the relative said. "You are just so strong through all of this."

As my mother later recalled the statement to me, she asked me with feigned curiosity:

"What choice did I have?"

We both knew the answer to that question.

The mistake people make when they look at you after you become one of the bereaved, after you become a survivor, is that they see you appearing to function and ascribe some lofty virtue to your efforts, not realizing that you are marshaling every available resource simply to appear normal while in their presence.

You're doing your work and taking the kids to soccer practice and getting groceries and attending Christmas parties because you have no other options—and because those things are necessary distractions that busy you between those many private moments when your heart explodes once again, and you fall apart in quivering fits and floods of tears and curses at God—and your voice making terrible sounds nothing other than grief can produce.

And this is the truth about those of us who are living with the loss of someone we love. However together or capable or steady we might seem or be able to project in the small sliver of time when you see us on social media or pass us at work or run into us at the grocery store—we are far less together, capable, or steady than you think.

Regardless of the sturdy facade we put in place, we are likely falling apart just out of sight. We are shattered and pissed off and paralyzed with pain, and we are weak enough to be knocked down by a song on the radio or the sight of their shirt hanging on the door. We're curled up on the bed we shared with them, or we're staring at the empty chair across from us, and we're as far from strong as we can be.

Because the reality of becoming one of the bereaved is that it isn't poetic and it isn't beautiful and it isn't instructive—it just sucks.

Yes, you're desperately making lemonade but it's always going to be more bitter than sweet.

No, we're not strong, we're grieving.

We are the people our loved ones are survived by.

And we're just trying to survive.

© 2020 John Pavlovitz

@John Pavlovitz
johnpavlovitz.com

Holly Richard

Trimming the Hedge

(One parent's journey through losing a child to brain cancer)

My mind feels numb; I look out and gaze at nothing in particular, wondering, not believing.

It's time to trim the hedge; I can see that it is overgrown.

The doctor said that my son has brain cancer. My son. My wonderful son who has really only started to live.

Brain cancer.

How is this possible? He is so healthy. Has always been so healthy.

An amazing neurosurgeon removes it all and I can breathe again.

I am swirling in a vortex of shock and relief. He's going to be fine. The doctor got it all.

What do you mean it comes back?

Why does he need all this radiation and chemo? Are you sure?

What do you mean it comes back?

My guts twist within me to see my son, my son, all scarred and scared.

This cannot be happening. I need to look away, think of something different.

The stress, the horror of it all makes my mind feel numb; I gaze at nothing in particular, wondering, not believing.

It's time to trim the hedge; through my tears I can see that it is overgrown.

It has come back. Those words echo through my head, bouncing back and forth like a sharp, jagged piece of metal.

The blood freezes in my veins and my breathing sounds like a car sputtering as it runs out of gas. I cannot eat, cannot sleep.

More treatment. This time, we throw "advanced" treatments at it. More scars, more fears.

What do you mean it's not working and there is nothing else that can be done?

What do you mean? What can you possibly mean?

It is not possible for my son to die. You cannot mean that. Do SOMETHING!!!!!

My heart explodes into little pieces like a glass vase thrown with force onto a stone floor.

My mind feels numb; I gaze at nothing in particular, wondering, not believing.

My eyes see but do not comprehend.

The six men carry a casket toward me as I stand wobbly on the grass near a freshly dug grave.

I know my son is in that casket, but I also don't know it; I can't know it.

If I know that he is in there, then all the Hopes I have ever hoped and all the dreams I have ever dreamt are also in there.

In a blur, fine words are said, hugs are hugged, the many kind people depart.

I am left, staring at the dirt, until eventually I reluctantly go, leaving. Leaving my dear son but now and forever never leaving him. Large and important parts of me are buried with him.

How now do I live without him, without all my best dreams, without a future, without any hope?

I now only have today. All I can do is pick up the enormous weight of my sadness and grief and go on, learning to be okay just to find meaning in little things.

But my mind still feels numb; I look out and gaze at nothing in particular, wondering, not believing.

Life goes on. It's time to trim the hedge; I can see that it is overgrown.

Time does go on. My heart remains bruised and in pieces. But I am aware that something has changed. Something I did not expect.

I am surprised by Love.

The love I had for my son in life continues to grow. How is that even possible?

If he is gone, then love ceases, doesn't it? But it doesn't.

The love is growing. I am sure of it. I can sense a stronger tether forming between me and my son.

Now I realize that he may be gone from this life, but he is obviously alive in another.

How did I not know that?

All that I loved about him like his sense of humor, his generosity, his courage continue to live.

Now I realize that the brain cancer only killed his body but did not, could not, kill his soul. The very best parts of him still live.

A bit of Hope returns to me; that long, anguished time after his diagnosis no longer grabs me by the neck, strangling me as it did. My heart starts to recover.

A springtime returns within me, producing tentative, pale green buds of Life and interest.

I can even sense there is a chance summer may come, and it will be time again to trim that hedge.

By Jana, mother of Aaron

Chapter 12
Grief, Grief, and More Grief

January 2020

It was the day the music died, the day the earth turned cold, the day when the world lost all color, the day when it had been a little over nine months without Derek. I woke up at 5:47 in the morning; he had passed at 5:48 a.m. I was still at times unable to process it, and then the numbness entered to give respite to my sheer panic.

Another friend responded to one of my "don't call me strong" rants, and she could imagine it as much as possible without having gone through the devastating experience.

I don't know how you do that. Faking normalcy is tough. I hear you about the music or songs. I know you get Derek coming through the piped in music in a restaurant or store. You see young men his age and you wonder why. I guess everything you are gets tested. We never want this to be us. It must feel like forever until you see him.

Holly Richard

I have looked out into the world each day, sometimes colorless and other times so colorful that the purple veins and red, thumping hearts are making their way through their day. So many intricate organs, right down to our bazillion cells, molecules, white cells, red cells, so much that goes on in the background to keep us alive and healthy. Derek was an organ donor. I was knocked to the floor again when even this was stolen from him and from me. This cancer, horrific, monstrous cancer. His handsome, strong outer casings, his beautiful insides, once so healthy that he could jump 800 feet out of an airplane with a 40-pound rucksack and land in a matter of seconds. His organs could have saved many, yet no one asked for them. The question went unspoken. Brain cancer and the one and only treatment method, radiation, took that away from us too. I have watched the news and have seen where someone who lost their precious person had that person's heart beating in another. I've mourned again and again, coupled with that misplaced, angry grief. Grief was so deep that it had no bottom.

Grief gets no respect in society, no recognition of how serious, debilitating and paralyzing it can be. Grief can mimic life much like someone having major surgery. The person is under the knife, pumped full of anesthesia but breathing, and the body is still functioning even though the person is unconscious. Never have I felt so uneducated about grief! How can we recognize that the bereaved, the grief-stricken employee, friend, or family member, needs more than a three-day recovery period? Mourning is more akin to heart surgery where a heart was dying. In the case of the bereaved, the heart is too sad and exhausted to keep beating. The infamous bereavement policy. Why is there a place for everything and everyone except for the grievers? When we are sick, we go to the hospital, when we are weary, we go to church, when we have a substance disease, eating disorders or other mental health events/needs, we turn to inpatient treatment facilities for respite, for medical attention, for access to life-saving resources like psychiatrists, social workers, and counselors. Yet when our precious person dies, no one wants to talk about it and we have nowhere to go.

Our loss is not acknowledged, not understood, and therefore nonexistent. We suffer in all types of ways. We experience darkness, pain, anger, numbness, excruciating heartache, panic, and anxiety attacks. The perception is that we will *get over it* and move on. Uh, no, we don't. We grievers need a grieving place to rest our broken hearts and broken dreams. We need someone to take care of us, to feed us, or to sit quietly with us. We should have access to grief counselors, chaplains, therapy dogs, to other people who know our pain!! Maybe this was what I was destined to do now with my pain, to create this haven for us grievers that no one can see.

I heard this analogy at one of my grief support groups. "We look normal yet are propelling ourselves in our invisible wheelchairs. No one holds open a door, gives a caring smile, because they don't see us; our disability goes undetected, unresponsive, unacknowledged; we suffer in silence." And I also need to kill brain cancer!!

Another piece of mail arrived addressed to Derek Ray Lemieux, another knife in the heart. I wrote "Deceased" on the envelope, underlined it 10 times, and added, "Return to Sender." Why can't the world finally realize that we lost someone with so much to give? How can they not know that my son is gone? The love of a child and a mother, his hug, a pat on the opposite shoulder so I look the wrong way. And he would smile and say, "I duv da momma." Why can't the world acknowledge he is not on this earth? What the hell!

I had just returned from my Tuesday grief support group where so many people were heartbroken. We were like ghosts until we got to the group; then we became visible. There I was. I could see myself and listened intently to others. I had come to finally find a softer way to accept different grief into my heart. This out-of-order death, the loss of a child, was so wrong, so unconscionable. My misplaced anger and grief were becoming more acceptable now, thank God.

Another member spoke at the meeting. We will call him Joe. He lost his wife of 63 years a few months ago. Could you imagine waking up every day for 63 years next to the same person? I am not sure how anyone could do that, but my Aunt Nancy and Uncle Fran did as well for 65 years and then passed away within ten months of each other. Forever they remain with two hearts tucked away into one soul. And there were so many of their children, my cousins, left behind who miss them every minute of every day, including me.

I was in a blank mode. I opened this laptop to share something I felt compelled to share, and then it left me like a caged cockatiel flying out an open window—gone! Oh, now I remember.

An image popped into my mind on my way home from my support group in Durham. It seemed like everything and everyone was in Durham—Duke Hospital, my grief support group and grief counselor. I had spent two months traveling between Raleigh and Durham every day, mostly early mornings into late nights, back and forth to see Derek. Listening to the radio on my drive home, I heard the Arby's commercial say, "Fish sandwiches are back for a limited time," and it took me back. I remembered Derek and me cheering to our fish sandwiches like we were raising Vikings' beer mugs. Lettuce and tartar sauce flew everywhere. I have a photo I took of us. Thank God I took a few pictures. I wished so badly I had taken more; other times I wish I hadn't taken any. It is what it is.

Chapter 13
The Broken Heart

January 30, 2020

I was talking earlier to Jana, the mothership of the Inspire website for the brain tumor community, sharing with her about the atomic grief bomb, the explosion and annihilation of one's soul after a devastating loss, then the aftershock. By the way, Jana is the only person who has permission to refer to me as strong. Her response was grief can be as serious as a heart attack.

Dear Holly,

Oh, you are most definitely strong. Exactly the very next day after you lost Derek, another woman lost her daughter (daughter was in her 20s) to GBM. That mother, because of all the stress of grief, eventually suffered a heart attack. (It was determined medically there were no blockages, so it was a stress-induced or more appropriately a grief-induced heart attack.) Because her intestines were deprived of oxygen for several minutes due to the heart attack, part of her intestines were damaged, so they turned gangrenous and died. She not only had to get back on her feet heart-wise, but she had to have parts of her intestine removed. She is continuing to recuperate and is now doing okay but only okay.

Holly Richard

Meanwhile, in a startling contrast, you have stayed on your feet and are engaged in fighting this disease head-on. Derek is, I have to believe, so proud of you for bravely weathering his terrible loss and defiantly not allowing this disease to take anything more from you than it did.

So, you are most definitely strong. And that's why I admire you and all that you are doing.

God bless you,
Jana

I started to find more opportunities to write to release some of this unbearable pain and suffering heart. This was from a half-day retreat with writing and yoga in September of last year.

At the Lake

I wait for you

I see you on my left

Walking beside me

Comforting me

At the lake

I wait for you

Then we see the ducks

Turtles on their logs

The cotton ball clouds

We look at each other

And smile

At the lake

I wait for you

To walk by my side

My son

I wait.

© *Holly Richard 2019*

Little did I know

Over this past year, my

Velocity driven son, would

Enter the sky and

Do the rest of his travels in heaven

Enter my place where

Mom is waiting with

Pride and open arms

To hold you, hug you, tell

You how much you mean to the world

Holly Richard

At a writing class sometime in February 2020, the prompt was to think of photograph and what it means based on who/what is in it.

The Photograph

I am thinking about one of my favorite photographs which was taken when my daughter Nicole was helping Derek with his homework at the dining room table at our old home in Waynesville, North Carolina.

I still have that table, and at an angle you can see some handwriting embedded in its surface.

Derek is watching intently, focusing hard on learning from his sister, whom he loves and admires. Nicole is looking proud and is also admiring her brother, whom she also loves and adores.

I think Nicole was twelve or thirteen and Derek around seven or eight in the picture. I believe it was around the holidays as I recall the tablecloth and, if memory serves, Nicole's sweater had a Christmas tree on it.

As I watch them, I remember how much I loved being their mom. I felt so lucky to have both a daughter and a son, two beautiful, healthy, loving children. I felt such hope and excitement watching them grow. What would they become; what would they do in this life?

As a child, I was denied the kind of love and protection, the stable childhood I wanted. But I was so committed to my children, their warrior mother, protector, and nurturer. Everything I had in my heart I wanted to pour out into theirs.

The photograph shows all the love I did pour out to them. I did my very best to love them unconditionally. I am in awe at who they have become. So proud I am to be their mom.

Now, this picture is also a reminder that half of me is gone. There is only Nicole left at the table. I feel her loneliness with mine.

The photograph shocked me back into where I am today, the loss of my precious son. Gone from this world way too soon. Brain cancer came from outer space, it seems. In four months, it took him from this life, from our world.

The photograph brought me back to when life was simple. I so loved simple. I could make happiness for them so easily. Trips to Toys R Us, the magic of that time when Santa Claus and the Easter Bunny were real, and the excitement of waiting for them to come could never tire me. So simple, so protected, so loved, so part of me and me so much a part of them.

Here is another writing class prompt which asked us to write a poem reflecting on "What the Living Do" by Marie Howe. This is what my pen put to paper.

Those Left Behind

Many times since you passed away, my son, I find myself now,

With mundane tasks of food shopping,

What was once a happy moment to look forward to weekly.

I pull into the parking lot at the grocery store,

A place I once loved to go,

And now I crawl out of the car,

Not wanting to go inside.

Holly Richard

For there were many aisles

With your favorite snacks.

I pass by the frozen sections

One by one.

Hot pockets, Baron's pizza,

The crustless peanut butter and jelly pockets.

On to the next,

Twizzlers, Swedish fish,

And, of course, rainbow Skittles and Reese's cups.

Then the next aisle,

Your favorite root beer, cream soda,

Gatorade

Followed by Red Bull and Monster.

It's amazing you had no cavities!

But I did take you to the dentist faithfully.

The Army looked after you from there.

And after nine years of service,

Home for good at last.

The new freedom you now had;

The menu of self-indulgence

Was endless.

How excited you were to

See me come home with

Special surprises of your

Favorite sweet tooth snacks.

Since you passed

I've left a few carts in the

Aisles now,

Unable to watch the items be scanned

Without your favorite surprises on the conveyor belt.

Now there are fruits & veggies and fresh

Produce to scan.

I look down at the floor

Until the beeping stops and pay the cashier.

She asks me if I found everything okay.

I glance at her;

She turns away.

I make my way back to

The dreaded parking lot.

I can't remember where I parked.

Minutes of wandering the lot

I find my car.

Throwing the bags in the trunk,

Wishing so much the bags were full of your favorites.

Holly Richard

As I close the trunk,
I remember once again
This is what the living do
Now that you are gone.

© 2020 Holly Richard

Another February 2020 writing class prompt was to write based on the inspiration of Roger Rosenblatt's *Kayak Morning: Reflections on Love, Grief, and Small Boats,* which is about the inability to be present among friends after suffering a death and how out of place one feels. My thoughts are shown below.

Maybe I Will Pray Again

In the heart of big cities, a host of enormously tall cylinders, giant pillars of pollution, spew their puffs of smoke out into the sky like my father's cigarettes as he blew the smoke into my face. He taught me how to make smoke rings with the tightening of the jaw, snapping outwards, mouth in a circle as you exhale the cloud of poison from your lungs, a perfect smoke ring. I was only ten.

When my children were little, I would blow into the bubble wand, filling their bubbles with my cigarette smoke and watch them in amazement; how much fun they had when popping those smoke-filled bubbles! I am not proud of that mommy moment, but I am grateful I was able to finally quit those cancer sticks many years ago. I am sure I have not escaped their residue;

it's just a matter of time. Cancer never dies; it invades, re-invents itself always.

I find grief quite similar: it affects everyone. I feel like the smokestack, giving off such toxins that all around me stare. "Surely she must get over this," I hear their voices say, but their eyes do not speak such harshness. It is me, my own tormented, damaged, sonless mother who watched her child be murdered by brain tumors.

I emit another black puff of smoke to the sky which I once looked up to for so long in faith. Now I look up with empty eyes, polluting the skies and those around me with my grief, hopeless, faithless grief.

I want the smokestack to close, to exhaust everything in it so the earth can live again, so I can live again, with hope for a sliver of warmth, a ray of light, when the smoke clears, and my eyes have color once again.

And then maybe, I will pray again.

© 2020 Holly Richard

Chapter 14
Sometimes There Are No Answers

February 6, 2020: after a decent workout at the gym

Grief is complicated because death experiences are so different yet can morph into one. It just depends on who you are, who your person was that you lost, and why your person had to die.

Grief support groups can specifically relate to the person who was lost or to who remains behind. There may be groups for grieving mothers or fathers who have lost a child, groups for children who have lost parents or siblings, groups for those who have lost spouses and so on. Grief is complicated both for the grieving person and those who love that person. Society as a whole does not have a means to acknowledge the magnitude of grief and has no clue what to do with grieving people.

Thankfully, in our society, we have a genuine love for our fellow humans and values that include caring for those who have suffered a loss. As a result we have established groups, workshops, art therapy, and other resources for children who have lost a parent, siblings whose sibling has died, a parent who suffered that out-of-order death of an infant, a child, or an adult child, and the widowed.

Then there is the *why* and what happened to that person you are grieving. Was it the baby not born or who was born but left this world so quickly—stripped from your arms in the hospital—or was it the little heart of a small child that a virus decided to infect, or was it your little one who closed sleepy eyes to dream and never awoke or the predator pediatric cancer? Was it a teenager in a car wreck or a young person who was poisoned by a substance that should not have poison in it, or was it an adult taken by the invasion of a tumor that started with one bad cell?

All these causes and losses are so varied, yet we, society, tries to link them all together like a barrel of monkeys. People end up letting go at some point, and some fall back into the barrel and try to crawl out again and again and again. That's because they eventually realize their grief, their loss, their person lived differently in this world and died differently. At the end of the day, those precious ones are gone from our physical presence, and that is our common thread. But the aftermath can be so diverse; therefore, grief is unique to each of us.

That part of the grief journey may be something we need to look into further. Why do survivors survive? How do we learn how to carry our person and inch forward with our person tucked ever so gently in our heart but not *move on*? In my short grief journey, thus far I have realized we do not even give grief a spot in the mental health oasis of life. It all leaves me baffled. Anyone who experienced grief knows damn well there is no shelf life to grief. It is forever on this earth with you.

Let's have a hard conversation about how we got to this place. Let's talk about why and how we lost our person.

Derek, my healthy son, was 27 years old, healthy one minute and taken from us in one hundred and twenty-six days. That journey of over four months is much different from what happens when someone receives the call from hell in the middle of the night to tell them their person has been taken. You who have experienced that horrific call know what that feels like. I do not, so I can only imagine it as I write. You hear that ring, and your heart feels like it will beat out of your chest. And the news comes. It cannot be true; he or she was just here. Your person or people are gone, just like that, in a flash of light, in one breath, *gone!* That kind of experience produces a whole different series of explosions inside one's heart and brain. It feels like one's soul has been electrocuted, obliterated in a second—no last hug, no goodbye, just nothing. Much different from my experience.

Was it a car wreck that suddenly took your person, an accidental overdose because a drug lord hid the poisonous fentanyl, or a terrible freak accident, an evil one-punch death blow, an eating disorder? Maybe there still is not an answer as to what really happened to your person. Or did your person take their own life because they could not see a way out? Regardless of the circumstances, guilt plagues us like a predator in the shadows. We are the parents and, therefore, *somehow* we believe we could have saved our child, but that simply is not true. Nevertheless, we beat ourselves up over and over and over again. The *would haves, could haves, should haves* shout at us all the time!

Then there is the horror and/or sheer panic. These emotions are so varied, and then they trigger other emotions and events. All these scenarios differ, yet all are the same because, in the end, our loved one is not physically here anymore with us to hug, to hold, to smell. There is no good way to lose someone we love so much.

What about the grievers who shared that special relationship with a soulmate, whether for a year or two or 60 years waking up next to each other, and now that person is no longer in this life? All the plans you had with that special someone disappear—whether it was planning a family, preparing for retirement and travel, time to visit with grandbabies. The one who remains behind in this life grieves for all the shattered hopes and dreams that were taken when that person died.

The grief is different in every situation, and the journey is unique to each person experiencing loss. Please understand: I am not comparing the grief from one kind of loss to another—just the opposite. I am simply asking questions, putting these scenarios out there. We have to keep talking about grief because society does not acknowledge it the way it needs to! We are all human; we share so many of life's experiences the same way, and we experience so many differently.

If we look at religions, the beliefs and experiences of Christianity, Islam, Hinduism, Buddhism, etc. are all distinctive and each has different experiences. We understand this and recognize those differences, so why do we try to force grief into just one category? Depending on who the one left behind is—a mother, father, sister, brother, child, spouse/partner, grandparent, cousin, best friend—grief can have a unique look and feel, yet people trying to help often do not know how to pivot from one to the other to support the person who is suffering. It is really hard to understand what to do in each specific situation. You get the point.

As a society, we seem to expect people who have swallowed an atomic bomb, been chewed up and spit out on the grief path, to piece themselves back together somehow. They're bewildered, disoriented, and in excruciating pain with a broken heart, but we expect them to crawl back and reintegrate into a world they no longer recognize. Back to work, back to life. Really?

* * *

On February 17, 2020, I went to writing class. It had been ten months since Derek passed away. Some days were unbearable. I wondered if this pain would ever give in enough to breathe the breaths needed to send oxygen to my brittle, worn, and torn body.

The writing prompt for class was "saying too much or too little." Here is what came out.

The Baby in the Cake

On Saturday, my husband and I attended an annual Mardi Gras get together with several couples that we do each year. Mardi Gras is a fun time to celebrate, wearing beads, eat good ole Louisiana famous foods such as gumbo, etouffee, and red beans and rice followed by the infamous king cake, the unity of faiths cake with different sprinkles of color representing justice, faith, and power. The baby inside the cake represents luck and prosperity.

Justice, faith, power, luck, and prosperity were some kinds of celebrations, but my grief turned it all dark. It went something like this:

Brain cancer? There is no justice; death is the only option. Faith? What faith could I have when my one and only son was violently taken from me? Power? WTF tumors, the most powerful cancer in America. Luck? Definitely no luck, GBMs are bad luck. Prosperity? That means flourishing, thriving. If you are a brain tumor, you are the most prosperous of all. Nothing can stop you; you are superhuman, undefeatable, spreading tumors throughout the invaded person despite an army of geniuses. Always a cell ahead. If you are a parent who lost a child, you are the opposite of prosperous; you are most likely…I digressed.

There is a baby tucked away in the king cake, a choking hazard for sure from my over-hyper, afraid mom perspective. The cake is cut into slices and whoever gets the baby hosts the next year's Mardi Gras. How I wish Derek was still tucked away upstairs, making his music, gaming, shopping for treasures on Amazon like he was before early December 2018. He was always there to greet me, anxious for me to hear the piece of music he was working on, updating me on his syllabus from his college at AIMM in Georgia. I wish I sat longer on that upstairs couch, asking him a thousand more questions on how he made all of those sounds instead of a few. I was often exhausted from the 14-hour workday, needing to get out of my work suit. Who knew those were the remaining days before the hospital awaited us, the invasion of the body snatchers?

* * *

On March 2, 2020, "Stocking Up" was the prompt in my writing class. My thoughts went like this.

Stocking Up

February 2019 was the final one my son Derek would be alive. This February was the first one he did not live in. A year ago last month, he was alive. The same is true of March. We celebrated his final birthday on March 26. This year, he would have turned 29. Then there was April; Derek lived 17 days in April 2019.

I have felt this uncontrollable urge to do things like brush up my resume and meet with people and friends I haven't seen since Derek became sick. I even entered a writing contest. I'm even considering seeking out ideas on how to start up a nonprofit for grievers, you know, those left behind.

I guess I am stocking up on all life's necessities as I prepare for the tsunami of emotions heading my way on the one-year anniversary of Derek's death. I did not realize just how much I was storing, but I certainly have been, kind of like my backyard squirrel, Sparky. He works on harvesting as he frantically digs little holes throughout the pine straw so he will have enough food to get him through the harsh cold. It's about survival. How will I survive this grief, the one-year anniversary of Derek's passing?

I will be harvesting too, like Sparky, collecting all of those edibles I can, creating stashes I can find when I am starved of hope to give me nourishment of something, anything to feed my famished soul that desperately misses my son.

I have a new appreciation for Sparky who used to swing from my bird feeder like a wrecking ball, flinging birdseed everywhere and scaring off the birds, lifting their wings to fly away. Sparky is just trying to survive the only way he knows how—by harvesting, stocking up to give him nourishment to get through the winter.

* * *

In March 2020, COVID hit our world and turned it upside down. America became dazed and confused, and panic started to enter our thoughts, our homes, bombarding us with the news. How could this pandemic be? Derek's 29th birthday would have been Thursday. I scrolled back through this book to read where we were a year ago on last March 26. Derek was alive, and we made it a day of celebrating as much as one can while in the hospital battling brain cancer. Four weeks later, on a Thursday, I was preparing for the ride to the cemetery, to Derek's grave.

If there was ever a mom jacked up about birthdays, it was definitely me. I celebrated my children's lives here on earth each year as if it were their first one. I hired a petting farm that came right to the house (true story, bunnies, goats, and horse rides, yes)! We had musicians, birthdays at Chucky Cheese, bowling alleys, you name it.

In 2020, I had to prepare for a different type of birthday celebration. I had no idea how to do that. Nor should I have. Nic would be with me; we were thinking we could get a couple balloons, write a special message on them to Derek and send them up to the heavens. That is not earth-friendly, but we did not know what else to do to get a message as high as one can.

April 10, 2020

Remembering the dreaded, most heinous, and unimaginable… in the ambulance with my dying son, heading to hospice, a year ago today. My mind pushed the memory off the track; my immense love for him pushed me back on the track. Off, on, off, on, off, on. There was a petition going around to identify what you call a parent who lost a child. The *out-of-order death* is different, not better nor worse than other losses, but it *is* different. It's your child—whether still in your womb or a baby, a child, an adult— and they are not supposed to die ever while in your world. But it happens over and over and over again. When a spouse loses a partner, she or he is a widow or widower. When children lose parents, they are orphans. When a parent loses a child, they are called "I can't imagine" people. We do not want to be called that ever!

In the "How Are You" chapter of this book is a list of what people need to be reminded of and educated on, what they need to consider before saying or doing something to be helpful to people in our situation. Those who have not walked in our shoes are at a complete loss as to what to say or do. And that is okay. There is no possible way you can imagine the depth of our suffering unless you have suffered the same loss.

I signed the petition started by one bereaved parent who is trying hard to get into the English dictionary the word vilomah to refer to someone who has suffered the loss of a child so we will have a name. A person who lost a precious child is a vilomah, which means "against a natural order." Back in 2005, Stacey Delaney used the name first in her great Ted Talk. This Sanskrit word expresses how unnatural it is for our children to precede us in death. This word represents our grief; we are vilomahs. (My spell check refuses to acknowledge this as a word, which is another punch in the gut; it really pisses me off.) My child died. If someone is an orphan or a widow, they have a name to acknowledge their unique grief. They can decide to defy or to relate to that designation, but at least they have a choice.

There also needs to be a name for those who have lost siblings too. I hear all the time "nothing can compare to losing a child." I agree *and* there is nothing that can compare to the suffering my daughter continues to endure after watching her only sibling, her only brother, die.

I was walking by the lake yesterday with a friend I met along this journey. She lost her son ten months ago, and I struggle to describe how he died. Accidental overdose for sure; he was poisoned, murdered. Her son had no idea the drug he took was laced with fentanyl, another F word with different meanings. Fentanyl was administered to Derek via a patch. The nurses were ever so cautious about removing it every 72 hours, writing the date when the new patch was changed out with a black Sharpie pen, wearing gloves because of its potency. It gave Derek relief from his intense pain of having tumors affecting every nerve. My friend's son was left on life support after that deadly dose of this poison drug. She had to see her son like that for five days and make the horrible decision to take him off life support, again letting go of her beautiful son, her only child. It is unfathomable. She had to make decisions about organ donations that could bring hope and save lives; parts of her son could live on in others. How many hundreds of thousands of our children and loved ones have to be murdered in order to get these monster drug dealers off of this planet?

I have gone through multiple stages of grief. They say there are five and now maybe six. I think there will be more, *a lot more*. The more vilomahs can be supported, their grief recognized by society as a debilitating event, when they can receive time off from work, not just a three-day bereavement policy, when society knows what *not* to say, when acute grief is acknowledged like we recognize those struggling with other acute challenges, there will be real hope, a place at the table in our society for those who are vilomahs. In April 2020, I guess I was approaching my acceptance stage of grief—at least in that moment. It can change quickly. The calendar does not lie, time has a way of gnawing its way through our concrete and cracking walls of our outer casings, letting me know, shouting it out from the rooftops, your son died a year ago on April 17.

I spent the one-year anniversary of Derek being gone with Nic,

Dave, and four pounds of crab legs to celebrate Nic's promotion. The news of her promotion came on the 16th, the day before Derek passed one year earlier. Is it a coincidence? I still challenge coincidences. Are they random things that just happen, or are they signs of some sort from someone we lost who is sending us luck, messages, something? I am curious. Celebrating Nic and her life and her promotion at work during a pandemic when the world has shut down was pretty incredible, and she is amazing.

On April 24, 2020, I was just reading how Valerie Bertinelli was dealing with the distancing during COVID and not being able to celebrate the birthday with her 29-year-old son Wolfie. Derek would have been 29 too. She said raising her son had been one of the highlights of her life, and she finally felt whole after she gave birth to him.

That is exactly how I feel about Nicole and Derek! The moment I became their mother, the chosen one, I finally felt whole too. I could love them with all the love I never received; I had double and triple love to give them; it had been swelling up in my body for years, stocking it all up like Sparky, the squirrel, and I felt like my mother love could start oozing out of my pores. I am still far from a perfect mom, but I was and still am unselfish. The mother love I hold in my heart is pure, not subject to any conditions, not determined by nor influenced by someone or something. This is the purest form of love, a mother's unconditional love for her child. I was and continue to be overprotective. Maybe that is why both of my children never ended up in the hospital like I did with broken bones, stitches, etc. Wherever my kids were, playing or at school, at an event, in their rooms, I would scour their environment like Arnold Schwarzenegger did in *Terminator*, like a robot, zooming in, scoping out anyone or anything that could be harmful. Is that TV stand sturdy; is that window too low to the ground; will they bump their heads on that; can they get their fingers stuck in those spaces? All these thoughts were constantly running through my head when they were growing up!

There are no words to describe getting through the year of *firsts*. I did my best to identify adjectives and analogies the best way I could in previous chapters.

Leading up to the first year without Derek, we saw an inordinate number of pop-up signs, much like highway signs when you are on a long, dreaded road trip, messages from billboards, 18 wheelers, rest stops, and gas stations. They are imaginary grief signs that start popping up, inviting us to remember when Derek did this or that, reminding us that it would be a year in *x* number of days since Derek passed. You get my drift. But during the year of *firsts,* there were no rest stops for a reprieve. Nada. Grief would not have it—at least not yet. I continue on the road trip from hell.

My grief counselor Mitzi and I talked *virtually* yesterday. It works and I can at least see her warm smile, her patient being and her understanding of the journey I have been thrown onto. I believe she must have been reincarnated as the angel of compassion and the angel of grief. In our session I asked her, "How can I feel both accepting that Derek is gone while being so damn angry because I know he is gone?" With the counting of the days, the flipping of the months on the calendar, the changing of the seasons and those damned pop-up signs and all of this happening in a pandemic—*I get it already*. I know he is gone—acceptance by exhaustion.

She processed all that I said, even with my profanity that adheres to other words and hijacks each word like brain tumors hijack cells. Mitzi proceeded with this:

"Holly, think of the seed that is under the ground. It has to somehow receive the water, the nutrients, and fight all kinds of hazards—dryness, wetness, rocks—and has to get the strength for the seed to crack open. Its sprout penetrates the ground, and, as it looks around, everything is charred, black, remnants of a massive forest fire. And there you are, like that seed rising among the ashes, making your way, reintegrating in a world you do not recognize, and in a pandemic."

These words aren't verbatim, but that was the gentle and loving message she gave me. Water fills the seed and activates the enzymes, the seed grows roots underground and then shoots upward towards the sun, and the shoots grow leaves and begin photo morphogenesis. She went on to say that for certain flowers, plants, and foliage to come back, there must be fires that burn, leaving blackness in order to make room for new life. (By the way, Mitzi is listed in my Warriors and Arsenals chapter.)

I had lost Derek after 126 days of living Gears of War, experiencing acute grief (out-of-order death acute) and feeling some form of PTSD. COVID-19 paused our world, killing so many including multiple people from the same family. People were dying alone; friends and relatives were left knowing their person would die without them there, that they would not physically be next to them to hold their hands as they took their last breath. My God, that is torture I cannot wrap my head around. I am so sorry for everyone living this horrific nightmare.

I was able to be there for Derek every day. I just cannot imagine. I think those bereaved because of COVID will have many more stages of grief that we have not even begun to acknowledge due to the additional trauma of the person whom they love more than life itself dying alone. How difficult being separated from a dying loved one must be, not able to kiss their cheek, stroke their hair, hold their hand, tell them over and over again they love them and are here for them. Instead, their person is in the

Holly Richard

hospital alone, and those who have COVID are hooked up to all kinds of machines while blue-gloved warriors and their arsenals try everything they can to save lives and hold their hands as the end nears while Facetiming their family to say goodbye as they take their last breath. I don't know how much more my grieving heart can take.

I poured a glass of wine. There are benefits that can help nourish the starving souls of people like us who lose their precious person. As in the ecosystem, a raging forest fire turns dead trees and decaying plant matter to ashes; nutrients return to the soil instead of remaining captive in old vegetation. I waited for those nutrients to enter my being. I had another glass.

Chapter 15
Coincidences and the Premonition

Coincidence 1: Derek could have gone from being stationed at Ft. Bragg, North Carolina, for the past six years to either Alaska or some other state on the West Coast or to Italy. Italy was where he went!! There, Derek had opportunities to work on making his music. He was becoming quite the musician and marketing man, all while traveling to 25 countries.

Coincidence 2: He bought a 2014 F Type two-seater, convertible Jaguar that was sitting in a dealership in Texas, sight unseen. The car shipped to our doorstep on a flatbed truck a week after he came home. Tada! Nic and I had never seen him more happy and grateful. I witnessed it with my own eyes and felt it all, goosebumps and butterflies, my heart swelling to the brim thinking, yep, I am his momma.

If this journey happened just six months earlier, these tumors could have invaded him in Italy, and if the tumors invaded his brain just three weeks later, he would have been in Georgia. But that wasn't the case, he was right under my nose where I was his guard dog. I was not going to let anything get in the way of his greatness and happiness.

And if his illness came a year later, with COVID-19, I can't even imagine the level of pain we would have felt having to be away from him through those months. The thought of it makes me want to vomit. As I can only imagine what brain tumor patients and their families are going through now when, if hospitalized, those patients have no one familiar with them. And all around them seeing COVID-19 patients and everyone in hazmat suits. In Derek's condition, what would have been racing through his mind with the sheer panic of having nothing familiar, no one to comfort him that he recognized, no one to help him eat his food when it arrived hot because there would not have been enough help to go around at times? There would be no one to sit and watch TV with him, to help him pee into that jug that hung by the side of the bed, to bring him peach shakes from Chick-fil-A or fish sandwiches from Arby's or chicken quesadillas from Taco Bell, no one to get him get into a wheelchair on a good day and get the hell out of that hospital bed and go outside to breathe in fresh air and feel the warmth of the sun's rays on his cheeks. No visitors, no friends and family who love Derek too. For COVID patients dying at alarming rates, what would it be like when their loved ones could not even have a funeral to gather in honor and memory of their person and celebrate a life well lived, to give and receive hugs that are a lifeline in this time of sorrow and despair? Nothing!!

There are so many coincidences. Do they add up to something more than meets the eye?

It was November 2018 right after Thanksgiving. I do not remember the exact day, but I recall all the conversation, word for word. It took me weeks after Derek passed away before my mind was able to extract that memory from my files. I was cooking dinner, spaghetti. Derek told me that he couldn't tell the difference between my sauce and the sauce he had so many times in Italy—whoa! I wondered what he was up to, but he said, "No, seriously, da momma, it is really good." He was leaning against the dishwasher, and I was cooking over the stove. His arms were crossed, he had his D-Rex T-shirt on, an expensive pair of jeans, and those black and red shoes that little did I know would be hurled across the hospital room a month later as he was whisked away for an MRI.

Derek was watching me cook, asking me about my day at work. His smile became an intense one and he proceeded to say, "You know, da momma, if I were to die tomorrow, I would be okay with that. I really would. I have been to places that rarely people ever get to go; I have served our country and played my music at a DJ Tour in Croatia. I made some songs and, if I were to die tomorrow, I would be okay with that."

I covered the sauce to simmer, walked over to him, and smacked him on his arm, saying, "What in the hell possessed you to say that, D?! You are 27 years old for Christ's sakes."

He gave me that coy smile and said, "I am not saying I will die, but if I do I am at peace with it all."

I paused. How I wish I had talked to him about death and dying that day. I would have asked him what he thought happened once we pass away. Did he believe in a higher power, in God, or that there was nothing? I think Derek struggled with the man upstairs, but deep down he had his faith restored in boot camp, where there was little to do other than running and more running, training and more training. It was hard! Going to see the chaplain on Sundays was his only escape from it all.

If I had that time back, I would have asked Derek how he would want to be remembered if he were to die and what type of funeral he wanted if he even wanted one. Did he want that gunmetal gray casket or to be cremated and his ashes sprinkled in some faraway land? How I wish I slowed that conversation down and really listened so I could have learned more about what his heart was saying. Instead, I did the avoidance and complete dismissal of death and dying thing.

What a gift he gave me that day. He was telling me how content and happy he was. He lived fast; what 27-year-old healthy son tells his momma that he is okay with dying? Did he know? Was he giving me a gift from his heart to my heart, a gift that would keep on giving, knowing how content and happy he was, knowing I heard it straight from his mouth, his voice, "Da Momma, I would be okay. I love you."

* * *

On March 16, 2020, I wrote the following passage in response to a writing prompt.

Cancellation

My subscription to my son's cell phone has been canceled. No more texts, phone calls, emails, or pictures from around the globe will come to me. No college graduation to attend, no watching him onstage as he mesmerizes an audience with his music.

No wedding to see him as he awaits his beautiful bride to be. No footsteps of a happy little one with Derek's big brown eyes looking up at me, the chosen and most favorite grandma of all.

It's all been canceled as the pandemic has done to our world. Everything canceled, church, school, weddings, funerals, restaurants, theaters—my God, everything. Cancer cancels everything in much the same way. It enters from the smallest places and spaces and, once inside, takes you apart, traveling through your human system, shutting down intricate parts one's body needs to survive.

Grief is like a shutdown, a cancellation of one's soul. Like an inward power outage, sitting in the dark, panicked, afraid, confused, discombobulated, utterly lonely and dreadful. But the inner power outage must be temporary; it must go away, but it does not. I must now feel my way around in the world, the colorless world. My mom subscription to my son is canceled until further notice.

* * *

May 3, 2020

I entered a writing contest in February right before COVID started. Of course, all three entries were on grief. Winners were chosen in April after COVID had invaded our world. When I was not chosen as one of the winners, I felt the talons of grief grab me again. Were my entries just too sad to publish, or was it not publishable material at all? Maybe I thought I had a chance, but what was I thinking. We were in a pandemic and this mom was wailing on her grief guitar to people who had their ears covered tightly, their hands cupped over them, to keep the grief noise from penetrating their healthy hearing ears. After all, in a horrific pandemic, let's not add acute grief to already scary times.

I read the essays that won—one about a car wreck, one by a daughter describing her mother's hands—they were all quite well-written. I think mine were well written too. I do think between the pandemic and my raw grief poems, it was way too depressing.

* * *

May 5, 2020: MRI

Why did I schedule an MRI on my hip today in the middle of a pandemic? It hurts and won't stop, and I have to walk the lake daily or I will go batshit crazy. All I know is I went and sat waiting for my name to be called. We were all masked, and I was pumping hand sanitizer into my hands and rubbing them together like I was ready to start a race or something. It was impossible to social distance in the waiting room.

My "thoughtful" grief personality took over, and I was both patient and polite. The woman across from me was sitting with her son. Of course, she was, and he was Derek's age; of course, he was. She had fallen and her son thought she might have broken her arm or wrist. As the mom whimpered as she spoke, I could see the worry in her son's eyes. He got out his cell phone and called his dad. He didn't answer, so her son left a message and said mom had fallen and they were at Urgent Care. There I sat, my thoughtful grief personality Googling what to do for a broken arm; I felt helpless that I could not help either of them. I wonder how often the frontline workers, nurses, doctors, police officers, firefighters, you know, those heroes, feel that helplessness. Especially now, now more than ever!

TOMORROW

Chapter 16
The Ugly Truth

My husband and I decided we were going to remodel our master bedroom. It was needed and would also be a distraction and a good project for me to oversee. So, one day, in my grief fog, I found myself wandering into a bath company's showroom trying to focus on choosing bathroom fixtures, not even sure how I ended up driving myself there. This nice lady from behind the desk smiled and asked if she could help me. As soon as I looked at her and our eyes met, I started bawling my eyes out. There I was, having a total meltdown in a bath store showroom in front of a bunch of strangers and surrounded by toilets and shower heads.

When I was able to catch what little breath I had to jumpstart the breathing process again so my lungs could fill back up with air and I wouldn't pass out, I apologized and proceeded to tell her the elevator pitch of what happened to Derek. Her eyes welled up with tears, and they began to trickle down her cheeks. She said she was so sorry; she has a son Derek's age, and she just could not imagine. I said I know as she passed me some much-needed tissues. Then, with her genuine and caring voice, she asked me if I ever read the book *Death Be Not Proud*. She went on to say it was a required read at her high school many years ago, and it was about a boy who died of a brain tumor. I went home and ordered the book on Amazon and read it.

The book was written in 1947 and published in 1949. It was a memoir written by John Gunther, an American journalist, after his son Johnny was diagnosed with glioblastoma at age 15 and passed away 15 months later at age seventeen. Mr. Gunther writes in the foreword, "*I write it because many children are afflicted by disease, though few ever have to endure what Johnny had.*"

I say all this to you, the reader, right now because it is chilling: The book had the same ending for Johnny in 1947 as we had for Derek in 2019, over 70 years later. Yes, 70 *damn* years ago. The same Tumorator tumor and the same outcome, devouring the precious life of one's person, taking his dignity and his sense of self until death.

I thought back to 70 years ago. I thought about the medical advances we have today. Thank God! It is absolutely amazing. The cutting-edge research (and a ton of federal funding) in the areas of prevention, screenings, treatments, and even cures for so many cancers that didn't exist 70 years ago. It is astonishing that you can take lungs from one person and put them in another, and they can breathe life back into someone's body. We can remove a beating heart from one human being and make it beat life in another human being. The same is true with other organs like the liver, kidneys, bladder, stomach, and intestines that can be transplanted from one person to another. It is truly astounding. Breast cancer patients now have an 84% survival rate of 10+ years. However, the brain, the organ that is the control center of the nervous system, well, you get the point. This isn't cancer shaming anyone. I am just stating facts. Society remains the same; those with the most popular cancers get the most money for research. The three percent of society who get the "bad luck brain tumor" diagnosis, well, sorry, not too much to offer. Over 70 years later, there is still a less than two-year survival rate for people diagnosed with glioblastoma, and top that off with a dreadful and cruel quality of life. Brain cancer funding for critical research treatments and a cure continue to be left in the shadows when compared to many other cancers. This must change.

Until Derek's diagnosis, although I come from a healthcare background, I didn't even know what glioblastoma (GBM) meant. If you, the reader, or someone you know has been diagnosed with a brain tumor, turn to the last chapter, *Warriors & Arsenals* to read ideas on what/who may be helpful to serve as your warriors along with the arsenal that may be needed to best support you or your loved every step of the way. The warriors and arsenals we had to put together for Derek, unfortunately, were assembled as we were being hurled onto the cancer battlefield, being shot at, cancer bullets whizzing by our heads, 24 hours a day.

Brain tumors are one of the deadliest and most debilitating forms of cancer and have among the fewest therapeutic options. Due to short life expectancy, long-term glioblastoma survivors are defined as patients who live longer than two years post-diagnosis. Yes, two years is a *long-term* survivor. Extreme survivors, yes, *extreme*, live for 10 years or more after diagnosis, and they comprise *less than one percent* of all patients (Bosn J Basic Med Sci. 2019 May; 19 (2): 116–124.). Who could have prepared themselves for this death sentence? The survival rate was six to 18 months at best for Derek with absolute shit for a quality of life to make matters even worse—if there were such a thing.

GBM threw Derek and us onto the cancer battlefield in an instant with no weapons, no shield, nothing. He was robbed of his young adult life, of marriage, children, a cat, a home decorated with all of his Army awards, all of his memorabilia from the 25 countries he traveled to, hardcore gaming with friends and people like Bubba Watson, being around the table at holidays, bowling and hanging out with his sister and friends. He didn't have the opportunity to plan an end-of-life trip to some place he had never been or to drink his favorite long island iced tea or tell us what type of burial he wanted. Did he want a military funeral with a gunmetal gray coffin with the American flag draped over it and TAPS playing or to be cremated and an urn placed on the mantle or to have his ashes sprinkled over Dubai where he zip lined down the tallest building?

So many questions lingered. Who did Derek want to give his precious possessions to? Who did he want to say goodbye to and be able to express his love with his own words? Who were the people he really wanted to see in his hospital room before brain cancer ambushed him and took his life, and who were the people he didn't want to see? Brain cancer was so vicious and violent that every organ in his body was riddled with cancer bullets. So much so that he and we were even deprived of giving any of his organs to save another and having at least a part of him live on in someone else's body. Nope, not with his kind of brain cancer and the blasting of radiation into his brain and spine every day for six weeks and the mountain of meds for 126 days that helped him to live and helped him to die. Robbed, robbed, and robbed.

I won't even try to go into the details about the science of the genetic makeup of brain tumors, clinical trials, treatments, etc. All of that is and continues to be done by the amazing, brilliant, loving, caring medical experts, professors of neurology, neurosurgery, researchers, oncologists, neurosurgeons; the list goes on and on of the army of brain tumor geniuses and advocates who have dedicated their lives to finding a cure. In the *Underground World Chapter*, there are real stories of people who have been diagnosed or whose loved ones have been diagnosed with a brain tumor and some discussions on what one does after that diagnosis.

Brain cancer needs to be talked about daily so people can be aware and know instantly what first steps may be, what to do, what questions to ask, what medical options are for treatment, clinical trials information, what financial assistance is available, and who and where the brain tumor experts are in this world. Where are the best hospitals that are equipped to treat these different types of brain tumors? No one is immune to brain cancer, and when it strikes its venom is fast, and there is little, if any, time to react and even know what to do to prepare for the unimaginable journey that lies ahead. Brain tumor information should be blasting on CNN, the *Today* show, on World News, Fox News, *Good Morning America*, radio, everywhere. Breast cancer, prostate cancer, pancreatic cancer, skin cancer, colon cancer, cervical cancer, ovarian cancer, lung cancer, kidney cancer, blood cancer (and I know there are more of the Cs), and they all can be awful and, damn it, brain cancer is awful too.

Brain cancer patients and families deserve clinical trials to give hope and treatments that are effective without the agonizing side effects many currently inflict.

- Did you know in 2020, nearly 700,000 Americans were living with a primary brain tumor and an estimated 87,000 more people were diagnosed with a brain tumor?

- Did you know there are only five FDA approved drugs and only one device to treat brain tumors?

- Did you know brain tumors are the leading cause of cancer-related deaths in children and young adults, ages 0-19, yes, little babies and children, for Christ's sake?

- Did you know brain tumors are now the leading cause of cancer-related deaths in men ages 20-39 *(National Brain Tumor Society (NBTS), 2020)*?

There is no cure for brain cancer, there is no prescreening

to detect or prevent someone from having brain cancer. There are few treatment options once you are diagnosed. Depending on the type and location of the tumor, some brain cancers offer little if any treatment at all not to mention that the treatments that do exist can be loaded with awful side effects. You wonder if you should have chosen that treatment in the first place, and that can leave everyone even more panicked, riddled with guilt, violently angry, and broken. Financially, it can drain the largest bank accounts in the world as the surgeries and treatments are so expensive. We must find a cure. We must get the federal funding that is long overdue so there is just not one treatment or not any treatment at all to offer someone who suddenly has a tumor growing in their brain, the nucleus of the human body. You can contact the NBTS and the ABTA to see how *you* can advocate for these changes to happen in the part of the world where you live.

Often, brain cancer, the platinum level cancer, is also commonly referred to as "bad luck" cancer and inevitably hands you a death sentence. It strips away a person's personality, cognitive abilities to walk, to talk, do self-care, to feed themselves and to go to the bathroom. When other cancers invade different parts of the body, a person can start trying to process in their brain about the cancer diagnosis they were handed with family, friends, medical professionals, etc. because the cancer is *not* in their brain. Once diagnosed with the cancer that is not in their brain, they can determine what treatment options they want or don't want, they can make key decisions on their own, using their brain to make choices based on their wishes. Because Derek's cancer invaded his brain, his ability to process the situation was immensely challenging and just as difficult for us.

In 2020, there were an estimated 1.8 million new cancer cases diagnosed and 606,520 cancer deaths in the United States. That is 1,660 people diagnosed and 69 people dying from cancer *every day*! Over 545,000 people have lost their lives to the horrible COVID-19 virus. In a year, our great country rallied around this deadly virus and attacked it with brilliant, warrior scientists and an arsenal that included all the expertise and money needed to find a vaccine to save our people. Cancer has been and continues to be a pandemic too, killing even more people each day, each year than COVID, yet here we are....

For so many people left in the aftermath, it is that blank stare into nowhere, wondering what in the hell just happened. Bereaved parents, children, siblings, husbands, wives, partners, grandparents, friends, families, and neighbors who have watched their loved one and themselves being thrown into the brain cancer mosh pit of hell, I am so sorry. You have had to watch a living nightmare unfold before your eyes with no pause button, no mute button, no sword to protect, to fight the monster killing your precious one, nothing. I am so sorry. The finality and the complete obliteration of one's heart and soul from losing your precious loved one to brain cancer is impossible to describe fully. There simply are not enough adjectives in the American language.

My hope is that your broken heart will be pieced back together as best it can. Although the heart will be of different shapes and pieces, and it will never be the same, it still beats for the love of your child, your loved one you could not save no matter what. I hope that you find a way to eventually begin to move forward with your loved one(s) tucked in your hearts. If you or someone you love is thrown into this new and painful reality, I pray there are people with you, walking beside you, and that they recognize you and *see* you. They may not know what to say or what to do

Holly Richard

(the *How Are You Chapter* in this book may help), and that is hard for us bereaved. Even when we are grief stricken and exhausted, we also have to teach sometimes and sometimes we have to learn to ask for help.

Chapter 17
How Are You?

If I did not include this chapter, I would have failed to do my small part in this crazy world. It is about what people should and should not say to a grieving person. People need to understand more about this, and it is hard because you want to do *something*, anything, to help and that is genuinely true. In full transparency, I had no idea either as to what to say or not to say until now. I am pretty sure I have said or done several on the list below. Also, know that I understand that we all grieve in our own way and own time. My suggestions listed below may not be the same for others who are grieving, and I get that. I do hope this chapter will help people stop and think in these terms. Although you may not understand, you can listen to yourself, and you can think a moment before responding or turning in the opposite direction when you see me walking in a grocery store, and the whispers say, "It's the momma elephant in the room who lost her child.... run!!"

Holly Richard

What should you not do then?

1. Do not say, "How are you?" I know this question jumps to
    the front of the line and shoves the words right out of your
    mouth. I have been guilty of this too! But be careful. Realize
    you are asking me how I am after losing my child from the
    WTF Tumor, after 126 days on the battlefield, after watching
    him take his last breath, then writing the obituary, figuring
    out what, where, and how to honor him, planning the funeral.
    How do you think I am? I have no clue.

2. Do not, I repeat, do *not* say, "God needed him more." Really?
    You are selfishly going to tell this to a mother and father who
    never got to take their baby home from the hospital and place
    their precious one in the decorated room full of Winnie the
    Pooh? Really?!

3. Do not tell me time will make it better. *Nothing* makes losing
    a child *better.*

4. Do not tell me everything happens for a reason. Are you
    serious? You think there was a reason for watching my son
    being attacked with brain tumors until his death? Really?

5. Do not tell me how strong I am. Oh, my God; please do not
    say that. When you have a choice to let your lungs fill up with
    water or hold your breath, you must make a choice, but it
    doesn't mean you are strong. You are surviving. And, besides,
    only Jana, the mothership, can say I am strong.

6. Do not send flowers. It is such a nice gesture; it truly is, but
    don't. Donate somewhere. Don't make me have to take care of
    the flowers, change the water, remove the dead blooms, and
    keep the live ones; that is more work than I can handle and
    is followed by guilt because you paid so much for them, and
    I killed them.

7. Do not tell me you know how I feel because you lost your uncle. I am not diminishing your loss. The out of order death of a child is different. It's an anomaly. Do not compare your loss to mine because then you pair your person with my person, and they are not the same, they did not live nor pass away in the same way.

8. Do not send joyous pictures of your happy, healthy family at the holidays (at least for the first year, please). I am mourning the death of my child who was robbed of ever graduating college, making it on the big stage, from his wedding, his children, his entire life. Just stop and think a minute.

9. Do not send me an Xmas letter detailing all the events of the year with travel, the aches and pains of getting older, visits from your adult children and grandchildren. Please wait at least a year.

10. Do not tell me getting back to work is a good distraction. Do you remember the game pong? That is what my brain looks like—black screen, darkness with a white ping pong ball going back and forth mindlessly as it cannot process the annihilation of my being. My heart is in a million pieces.

11. Do not ask me what I like to do so you can help me find a hobby. Really? Are you kidding me?

12. Do not ask me questions about the doctors and why they did this and not that or grill me about justifying the medical treatment and care. You are telling me I did something wrong, adding more guilt and panic. Are you a cancer doctor?

13. Do not tell me that if it happened to you, you could not survive. Gee, thanks, more guilt that I am not in enough pain to kill myself. That would be easy. Dealing with this out of order death is suffering at its finest.

14. Cards are thoughtful. When you lose that person that you love so much, it is quite normal to feel anger at its finest, pure, raging, and sometimes misplaced, ugly anger. You just can't help it. I have met many vilomahs who agree. Faith is challenged. How could my loving God allow this to happen to my loved one? Also, understand there are grievers out there who do not believe in a God, so I would make sure sending religious cards would be comforting to your person and not make them angrier.

15. Sending food is so thoughtful; it really is! But don't unless they tell you that would be helpful. Otherwise, donate or make a sympathy gift to a local charity. Stomachs are in knots. Diarrhea and constipation along with nausea and vomiting make it hard to decide what to eat. What you think would be something everyone would eat may not be helpful for those who are grieving. Some people also struggle with eating disorders. A gift card to a local grocery store could work. If your person is okay financially, donate and send the person a note that you did it in memory of their loved one.

16. For a while, don't expect your person to be the sharp thinker they were. In grief, memory is affected; the ability to remember dates, directions, and events is on pause. Please don't say, "Don't you remember I told you that yesterday?" Really? I can't tell you what I did an hour ago. My child died, so I don't remember, god damn it!

17. Don't abandon ship. Don't avoid or stop calling because it makes you uncomfortable. If you really want to help your person, then get comfortable with being uncomfortable.

18. Don't say you will see your person again someday. That does nothing for me when I just watched him die a vicious death. I want to see him *now*. This can't be happening!

19. Do not avoid talking about the person's deceased loved one. Yes, it will make me cry and that's okay; I lost my child. Not talking about him hurts badly; not speaking his name dismisses him as though we forgot him. Talking about him keeps his memory alive. Be comfortable being uncomfortable.

20. Do not say "happy holidays" at least for the first year, and then do a re-check on each holiday thereafter. Do you realize your beautiful children are home with you and my son is buried in a cemetery? Please think a minute. Maybe you can say something like, "I don't know what to say. I wish I knew what to say but I don't. Can I give you a hug? I am so sorry and am here if you need me." Something like that is more helpful.

21. Do not send me happy text photos of your grown children at Christmas when I just lost mine! Really, wait at least a year or two unless I ask.

22. Do not refer to my loss as "unfortunate." Really?! Being turned down on a promotion or breaking a mirror is unfortunate. The loss of a child is annihilating.

23. Don't say I had the "luxury" to live close to the hospital and didn't have to travel. We were grateful, but *luxury*—wtf?! There is no luxury in watching your child die. My God, people!!!

24. God forbid you had to experience the excruciating pain of losing a child. Do not tell anyone else who just lost a child and is grieving that "it only gets worse, sorry to say." OMG, really?!

25. Don't tell me at least I have another child; it dismisses the loss of my one and only son!

26. Don't suggest how I should honor the death of my son. It is

grossly unfair to put another guilt trip and another item on my already forever to-do list. Like what do I do with my dead child's clothes, possessions, his car, his bills? Then for someone to throw on to that, "Oh, let's honor Derek with random act of kindness to a stranger." I do that many times a year, and, frankly, do what you want to honor your person, but don't tell the grieving person how you think it should happen. You haven't lost a child, so stop it!!

27. Books are a nice gesture, but don't send them. Just because you think it would be good for me to read and love its message does not mean it will help me or that I will read it. Books to read are yet another item you have given me to add to my growing and grieving to-do list.

28. Miracles: I believe in them, and I also know how painful it is when people tell me about the miracles of their person and how it all came together, and they are no longer sick, and their person is doing wonderful. It is not that I am not happy and relieved for you, but it does make me internalize all that Derek went through and wonder why he wasn't given a miracle. *Why?*

29. Lastly, consider the words you are choosing and their meaning when trying to console a grieving mother or father. Before you see the person, say your words out loud if you need to. Hopefully that will allow you to hear words that are hurtful and realize that would *not* be a good thing to say!

So what can you do?

1. Some people feel they need to say something for all the right reasons, but nine out of ten times it only adds to the anger or pain a grieving person is dealing with. It's okay to say, "I don't know what to say, and I am so sorry."

2. You can say, "I am so sorry for your loss."

3. You can say, "I do not know what to do to help. Just know I can be there anytime if or when needed."

4. Movie tickets may be useful. They can be a distraction when the gut-wrenching moments leave for a couple hours, and the brain fog creeps in. Other people may think, *really? You think I could go out to a movie?* I am speaking for myself. Movies were a respite where I could sit and just be in another place other than home. Of course, until COVID invaded our world.

5. You may offer a gift certificate for self-care for when we can hopefully manage to do so. In my opinion, a massage is critical to getting the knots of hell out of your neck and shoulders.

6. Be patient. I am no longer the same person I was before Derek's passing and will never be again. Things I may have enjoyed doing in the past, I no longer do; former pastimes pale for those who grieve deeply.

7. Numbness to what is happening: Be aware that I will do my best to empathize with you when you've experienced sadness or pain, but my heart is broken. As a result, I may come across as uncaring because I am caught up in a world of grief. I am not unsympathetic. It is just that I cannot carry your pain along with mine right now.

* * *

I wrote the following in response to the May 11, 2020, writing class prompt to express what "I appreciate." This was hard at first. After all, when you watch your child die, "appreciate" sounds more like the screeching noise of digging your fingernails into the chalkboard and slowing dragging them down to the floor.

I sat in silence, a blank slate, empty. Then a flicker passed through my mind. I thought how fortunate I had been able to take this writing class, to step away from work, and throw myself completely into the grief pool because my husband supports me. He loves me. He really *loves* me unconditionally!

I Appreciate

I appreciate all you do during this pandemic as you often go unnoticed, yet you work harder than anyone I know.

Seven days a week, looking after our state's most fragile people, ensuring inclusion for everyone.

I appreciate the long days you give, yet you have the patience to then turn to me with a loving smile even when I cannot smile back through my pain.

But I notice.

I appreciate how calm and nonjudgmental you are, unshaken by the earthquake unfolding under our feet in a turbulent and judgmental world.

I love you, DJ, my adoring husband. I appreciate you. xoxo

* * *

On Memorial Day, May 25, 2020, we visited Derek at the cemetery. There were no words that day. Mind numbing.

I was unable to come back to this book, my beast, until July 14. During that span, I made a few new friends on the grief journey, mothers who had lost their sons in all sorts of horrible ways; there is no good way to lose your child. I also joined Helping Parents Heal, a Facebook group where we share our broken hearts, our tired souls, where we post how beautiful our children are and ask, "Why, how could this be my life?" We share our thoughts and feelings on the grief merry-go-round:

I don't want to live.

How do I live without my son/daughter?

I can't breathe.

I am nothing.

I am broken.

The grief carousel circles endlessly.

I could not join this group for some time. I was not ready to see more beautiful children gone from their parents' arms. It took 454 days, 12 hours, and 53 minutes to finally join the group. Maybe surviving for that long is why I was able to nudge my way into the group. After enduring the year of "firsts" without Derek, I started the downward slide into the agony of defeat. No matter how long I climbed or how much I did anything, Derek passed away that day. After 454 days, acceptance of some sort happened for me. I had to accept it, so defeated, feeling like a failure of a mother who couldn't save him in the physical world, and I couldn't bring him back from wherever he was, which I hope is heaven. I still grappled with the anger and felt that there was a conspiracy that somehow, someone or something wanted me to suffer.

My daughter, my beautiful Nicole. For those of you who are familiar and know someone who is suffering from an eating disorder, it is another monster that threatens the lives of millions of people, my child included. I felt myself much more consumed with anxiety, worry, and fear, my heart racing like a mouse being hunted by a cat. I am a mother of two with one in heaven and one on earth. My precious Nicole has been fighting and fighting and fighting. Then she had to watch her brother, her only sibling, go through the tormented brain cancer gauntlet. She was such an amazing warrior for her brother. She knew when it was her shift, when she walked into that hospital room, if things were not right. She would start organizing the troops at the hospital so we could get things to be the best they could be. A chip off the ole block for sure.

Did you know that eating disorders are among the deadliest mental illnesses, second only to opioid overdose? Did you know that 10,200 deaths each year directly result from an eating disorder? That's one death every 52 minutes! There needs to be a whole lot more done for the eating disorder community. And by the way, mental illness is nothing to be ashamed of. It is a medical problem just like heart disease and diabetes. My God, can we recognize the need for funding and support for brain cancer and eating disorders, *please*?! All I ever wanted was to be the best mom I could be, and, oh, my God, to be a grandmother. Now that I have been schooled in motherhood for 36 years, I would be an awesome grandma. To look into the eyes of your child is heaven, and to look into your grandchild's eyes, well, that must be like heaven with twinkling stars, fireworks, and rainbows.

I could not bear to lose my beautiful daughter, my only child here on earth. How unfathomable to even think about it, but I cannot help but do so. I fear the looming last knife could still be out there waiting for the final stab on the heart that is just now growing a ring of cushion around its gaping hole. Where the cushion has some give, it is bruised really badly, but sometimes it can absorb the rapid fire of grief and loss. Could I become childless here on earth, stripped of my motherhood title by brain tumors and eating disorders? I was most proud of being a mom and worked at it every day of my life for the past 36 years to be the best. I am so afraid...

Upside down sky

Yesterday, October 26, 2020, when walking the lake, I noticed the reflection of the puffy clouds and light blue sky mirrored in the lake, the clouds floating along at a good pace. It reminded me of what grief can feel like. Having solid ground, gravity, and the ability to put one foot in front of the other means the world is okay. When the sky is upside down, how can someone put down one foot? Your foot would disappear and lower itself through the cloud, and the rest of your body would go down with you. The empty flopping in your stomach, your heart racing, feels like there is no bottom; you keep descending into nowhere.

Chapter 18
Flashbacks

As of February 10, 2021, I had been having some symptoms for a few weeks that needed an inside look, so my gynecologist ordered a CT scan with and without contrast at the imaging wing of a nearby hospital. I had to be there at 8 a.m. to get it done. On my way to the appointment, I had a flashback to driving Derek to the same hospital on December 12, 2018, at 6:30 in the morning. I remembered what he was wearing: his favorite jeans, his Oakley hat. I recalled the confused look in his eyes, his pale skin, and him trying not to puke in the bag between his legs. I remembered us walking in the same front entrance of the hospital that I entered that morning. I replayed the scene of us standing at the ER desk, Derek pulling out his Gucci wallet with the red snakes, presenting his ID and insurance card, and off we went to the back as we waited to be seen. You know the rest of this story.

I turned to the right and followed the signs to imaging. The walk felt like it took forever, and my eyes shifted up and down, left, right, and straight, and these motions repeated. I remembered the colors of the flooring, the shades of the square patterns in the upholstered furniture, the pigment on the walls. I remembered it all so vividly. It was the same hospital I took Derek to when he was throwing up and we thought it was a bad sinus infection.

I made it to check in and was greeted by a kind lady. Then I waited to be taken back. It was quiet just as it had been on that early December morning in the ER when I was relieved Derek could be seen with no wait. The technician came to greet me and walk me back to the CT room. She was wonderful. I was not sure of her credentials, what her true job title was, but she was caring and patient. I felt at ease as I knew she would make administering the IV in my vein to start the contrast as painless as she possibly could.

As the needle entered my vein, I looked at my arm and saw Derek's veins, covered with his sleeves of tribal tattoos, each one having a special meaning to him. I remembered a couple of occasions in the hospital with Derek when I noticed his arm was swelling terribly because the needle was not all the way in his vein and fluid was leaking out, making his arm swell. I found the nurse, and she quickly adjusted the needle. In my mind's eye, I saw his swollen, tattooed arm as I watched the needle enter my vein. I fought back the tears. The needle went in smoothly, and I was relieved. Derek had so many needles put in and taken out of his arms, hundreds if not thousands of times. When he was in hospice, little needles were placed so gently throughout parts of his body to give him the medicine needed to aid in his transition from his life to take his last breath peacefully. Transitions Life Care was our last stop on this earth with Derek. The hospice workers were all so special, angels of calmness and kindness.

I could process all that was happening during the imaging because I did not have a tumor swelling in my brain. I could think and comprehend; I got explanations for what was going to happen each step of the way, and I understood it all. While I lay there on the table as it started to slide me under the CT scan, I stared at the ceiling. I could feel Derek there with me. I wondered what was going through his mind during all of his treatments. Derek had so many different tests, treatments, IVs, injections, bladder scans, head scans, everything scans. Many of these he did not understand and couldn't process what was happening. Many times, he was in so much pain with every move or given pain meds to get through the procedure only to wake up in a tube, panicked and hyperventilating. It was awful. Other times, we were so relieved and grateful when we were able to get these things done relatively painlessly and with as little stress as possible for Derek.

* * *

On March 9, 2021, I had a dental appointment.

"Let's X-ray that tooth," the muffled voice under the COVID mask of the pleasant assistant uttered, trying to show her kindness, making her eyes bigger so I could feel her gentleness and caring for me having to be in the dentist chair. "Bite down and hold it for 30 seconds; okay, Mrs. Richard?"

I heard the machine scan my jaw, and the humming noise started. The noise was a trigger for my trauma, and there I was in the past again, watching Derek's chest rise and fall so rapidly, his frail, thin chest emerging out of the hospital gown, up, down, up, down so fiercely fast on the radiation table. His eyes wide as saucers with a big black circle painted in the middle of each saucer.

The humming continued, and so did my flashbacks: Nic and I were in the waiting room at Duke, praying Derek's MRI would go well, that he would remain calm and sedated enough to get through a 40-minute head and spine scan, lying still on his back, strapped to the board, to determine if the radiation was having any effect on shrinking his tumors. I told Nic to go home; we both had had a long day at Duke, and the hospital was running behind on getting to Derek, which made my anxiety even higher. *The longer the wait,* I thought. *It's getting too late. The longer the wait; it's getting too late.* Over and over inside my head, the words repeated like a deranged mother goose nursery rhyme. The longer the wait, the less potent his medicine cocktail would be. This scan was so important. We prayed the radiation was working. I was relieved that Nic went home; she was spared one of the many living nightmares and the sheer terror of watching Derek in the most pain I had seen him in since we arrived. Nic had seen her brother in so many scary situations already; it broke my heart as I watched her suffer as she helplessly viewed her brother's suffering. The only thing worse in that moment would have been if she were watching all of this unfold right now, the wound to the bone horrific.

The radiation team carefully moved Derek from his hospital bed, gently lifting him onto the MRI board. His eyes widened, his heart pumping, and he screamed so loud that it almost brought me to my knees. "He needs oxygen; get the oxygen," one tech yelled. I start shouting, "And get the Dilaudid into his arm *now*. I beg you, please."

Derek was grunting, his nostrils expanding like they could breathe fire; his oxygen levels had dropped to 40%. I was going to hurl right there. *No, stop it; calm down,* I told myself.

"Derek, I am here. Just try to breathe, okay, sweetie? They are getting you more medication; hang on, D; please hang on."

The needle went in a couple of minutes later, his chest started lowering, thrusting his upper body less high, less low, and oxygen levels started to creep back up. How was this all happening; how was this real? A few weeks ago, we were shopping on Black Friday for furniture for his apartment in Atlanta. Now we were in this living hell. What in God's name was happening to my Derek?!

I heard the dental assistant saying, "You are all set," and I left.

Chapter 19
The Underground World

In the underground world of the brain tumor community, there is a website from the American Brain Tumor Association (ABTA). It is an online community support website, *Inspire, www.inspire.com*. There you will find the mothership named Jana, and she is truly just that. She is the one who can handle the landings of heavy and broken hearts day in and day out on her vessel. She gives all she has to help the dazed and confused, the panicked and exhausted, the hopeful and the hopeless who have been face to face with the brain cancer beast. I am sharing below just a few of the hundreds of writings over the past eleven months of anonymous people in this brain tumor community who have found themselves in the underground world. This is to give you, the reader, a sliver of a glimpse into our world so you can realize that brain tumors are invading peoples' brains every day, and they do not discriminate. Please note the stories below have been modified to exclude any personal information and *Inspire* has approved.

I start with one of Jana's entries, describing the mangled destruction from brain tumors that took her precious son Aaron and the humanness she has found. There are thousands of others who live this hell every single day along with Jana, the mother of

Aaron, Joe's mom, Mary Ann and me, Derek's mom. It breaks my heart there will be thousands more if drastic change is not taken to adequately fund brain cancer research and critical clinical trials and treatments.

* * *

Dear everyone,

On the one hand, it seems right that there is no word in English for it. On the other, the absence of a name is a cruel reminder that fate has dealt some of us the most unspeakable blow: the loss of a child.

I knew what I was when my father died. I was an orphan. When friends sadly lose a spouse, they are instantly known as widow or widower, a name derived from the Sanskrit word for being lonely or solitary.

But what—or maybe more importantly—who am I after my dear and wonderful son has died? Some say, once a parent, always a parent, but that's just a cheap and easy platitude. Try telling that to a bereaved parent on Mother's Day or Father's Day or Thanksgiving. Try living in the empty shadow of brain cancer after suffering every mind-etching step of the journey from diagnosis to the funeral of one's child and beyond. Only after one sees the disease's unquenchable desire to rip life apart from its full bloom and potential can one fully appreciate the raw, evil destruction of brain cancer.

And so I sit here today, Mother's Day, nameless and bereft of my precious son. Instead of my son, I have a room in which I have a chest of keepsakes—his house keys, his favorite jeans, his favorite T-shirt, his computer keyboard, his various certificates of merit from school, photos and, oh yes, a growing pile of his mail received since he died, unopened and preserved with my irrational, pretended hope he is just on some secret foreign excursion somewhere and will return someday to open his mail.

I am sure that from the outside, I look whole and normal this Mother's Day, and I will smile graciously at the store clerk who wishes me a happy Mother's Day, but inside the pain and sheer weight of his loss is a reminder of all his preciousness that was lost.

So, what am I really called now? I think I may be called *hammered into awareness.* Why wasn't I aware of the losses being carried daily by so many people around me who had lost their children years before and who, after I lost my son, suddenly came out of the woodwork in large numbers? Why did something so terrible have to happen for me to have a better understanding of the fragility of even a healthy child's life? Sometimes, when I encounter a frustrated mom yelling at her pack of unruly kids in the grocery store, I want to walk up to her and clue her in that every minute of the lives of her children, however loud and out of control they may be, are gifts that can be snatched away in an instant by cancer.

Why did it take my son's death to really hammer through my stubborn head that the control we think we have over our lives and the lives of our children is paper thin and that, in reality, we live on an edge with constant uncertainty? Why did it take my son contracting and dying from GBM before I really saw that we are all one big family and that all of us are bound together in this constantly changing, sometimes beautiful, but sometimes cruel life?

I guess it took my son dying for me to have the clarity to realize that the name we all really get through our common challenges is not *orphan* or *widow* or whatever you call someone whose child has died. The name we get is, simply, *human*. Our struggles are universally human. Our journeys are across paths well beaten by other people who have gone before us.

However, it remains that we are the only species with the ability to make the choice of what we do with the suffering and loss we experience as individuals. I have learned that when we choose to accept the burden of our fears and pain and not deny them and when we muster the courage to acknowledge we are all just travelers in a temporary wilderness of uncertainty, a strange paradox emerges.

The very same darkness that hovers over the waters of death also holds the key to our healing. In supporting each other through our common heartaches, the fixation we tend to develop from what we experienced starts to chip off, and we have become strengthened enough to endure even the worst this life can throw at us.

This sort of healing happens not from what we receive and keep but rather what we share and give to others, even as we are hurting. The paradox of dealing with the intense challenges and heartaches of brain cancer is that, when we lift something to give to another, it is we ourselves who are lifted from the misery of this disease and we who diminish its dark powers over our lives.

With that, I lift my compassion and concern to those who have lost or may lose anyone to this disease and pray you will find healing and peace in your struggles.

Jana

* * *

Dear Jana,

I don't know the pain of a loss of a child, but I do know the pain of losing my wife to GBM. While different, I imagine the pain we feel is similar.

I, too, have asked many of the same questions you are asking yourself. Not so much the question of why this happened to me, but what now? I'm sure your life was as wrapped up in your son's as mine was in my wife's. Then, when the cancer came, we got to have a front-row seat in watching their demise. Extremely painful.

I hope you don't mind the ramblings of an old widower, but I will share with you some things that have helped me through this time. You mentioned the awareness you now have of others and the pain that is all around us that people are going through. Like you, I don't know where my head was before my wife got cancer, but my awareness and compassion for others was not what it is today. Maybe I was just too caught up in my own life to really care or take the time to care as I should have. So, when I look back over the events of the last few years, I search for any good that has come from it and find that I am a changed man, a better man. I value relationships more. My antenna goes up when I hear of trouble, particularly cancer in the lives of those I care about. Because of what I have gone through, I am able to help/comfort others in a unique way. I am thankful for this newfound awareness. I am amazed when I find out the storms in life people all around us are going through. Everyone is dealing with something.

The other thing that has happened is that I am finally figuring out a way to deal with the pain of her loss. There are some days I really have a hard time with it and shed a bunch of tears. During one of those episodes a few months ago, I came to the realization that the hurt and tears meant I still love her. I wondered, if I quit crying and feeling the pain, would I no longer feel love in my heart for her? If that's the case, then I will accept and choose to have that pain in my life so that I can always feel the love too. So now, when the tears come, and I miss my beloved, I cry out to God and thank him that I can still feel the love I have for her. I dunno if this makes sense to anyone but me, but there it is.

I heard an interesting story the other day that I will share.

I heard a story about a painting contest promoted by a man who sought the perfect picture of "peace." The artists were told to paint whatever they felt would portray peace. Some artists painted serene landscapes with sunsets and fields of beautiful flowers. Another painted a still, quiet lake with a reflection clear as glass. Each was amazing and beautiful, but when the winner was unveiled, everyone gasped in disbelief. The title of the winning painting was "Peace in the Midst of the Storm."

At first glance, the painting looked anything but peaceful. Black clouds and lightning covered the sky. Waves crashed down a jagged rocky hillside with raging waters below. How could this possibly be called peaceful? However, a closer look at the painting revealed that just beneath the raging waterfall, a little bird with her nest of chicks was tucked underneath the edge of a rock. In the midst of the cataract, lightning and wind, this little bird found a sanctuary, a safe place to rest with her brood, a true portrayal of peace.

Jana, I hope you and I and others on this site who have lost a loved one to this vile cancer can find peace through the storm. I pray for rest for your soul.

* * *

Another victim of brain cancer wrote in, and the mothership once again gave her love and straight from the hip thoughts. You never have to guess; Jana just knows.

Dear friend,

After reading your message, I wanted to crawl under the covers too and have a good cry with you. I lost my son to GBM, so I know what this disease can do and how much it can rob from our lives.

As one mother who has been through this madness and made a point of probably tripping into every pothole along the way, I will tell you that I doubt diet, exercise, and trying to be happy will work for more than maybe 15 minutes. That just sounds like putting lipstick and a dress on a gorilla to me.

If you really, really want to control what this journey can do to you emotionally, you are going to have to figure out a way to be of service to others. What happens to us when our children have GBM is that every thought and every emotion becomes hijacked, leaving us prey for forms of instant insanity and depression. The only way I ever found to diffuse its power and keep my head about the water line is to be busy being concerned about other people. Other mothers have told me the same thing.

That's the secret—you do not try to cover up or suppress all your overheated emotions. They are there and aren't going anywhere. If you try to suppress them, they will only pop out in some other part of your life, making a mess of that part of your life too. The best thing is to transform your emotions and re-channel them into something constructive.

You don't need to do anything as dramatic as the lady who started Mothers Against Drunk Drivers. You can do smaller things like organize women to knit hats and blankets for newborns at the county hospital. Maybe there is something you can do to get involved with other parents who are dealing with bipolar children.

I know things are tough right now with the COVID-19 restrictions, but there is probably something out there that desperately needs your skills and experience. Anything where you are helping others and keeping your mind off your own bona fide concerns for a while will help you stay on the right side of the covers and will allow you to have the strength to be there for your son who has the GBM when he really needs you to be there for him.

I am so sorry you are going through this, and knowing your son has a fever is a frightening situation on top of everything else. I hope you can use some little bit from this message to make things easier on yourself and your family.

Jana

* * *

My husband is now on inpatient hospice care. He was diagnosed with GBM and had resection surgery. He was doing okay during his six weeks of radiation and chemo. However, he had *many* setbacks. Without going into all the details, here is a list of reasons he was hospitalized:

1. He needed a shunt to drain fluid from his brain.

2. He had large blood clots in his legs.

3. He needed shunt revision due to clogging.

4. He had intestinal problems.

Once at home he was on *heavy* doses of steroids and blood thinners, took his five-day regimen of chemo tablets, and started Avastin. The fifth and last time he went into the hospital was because he didn't want to get out of bed for two days; he fell (not hard); he was *very* weak, was completely anxiety ridden (he's on Xanax and Zoloft) and had some confusion.

I finally called an ambulance when he couldn't get up at all. From there it was all downhill. He has terminal agitation, meaning he pulled out his IV, couldn't completely void his bladder, and tried to pull out his catheter, took off his gowns, pulled off his hospital tags, stopped eating and drinking, and now cannot communicate. He is constantly picking at his bedclothes and taking off his adult diapers. They had mitts on him and other restraints. They did every test one can think of, and there is nothing to treat medically anymore. His tumor hasn't even grown, so I don't understand what exactly happened! The doctors say all of the above could be contributing to his delirium and death.

Now it's all just comfort care, meaning medication to treat the agitation and keeping him clean. He is staying in the hospital because he's a danger to himself, and I can't be with him there. The one silver lining is inpatient hospice care is completely covered by Medicare. Of course, I feel guilty about not having him at home, but everyone on his team of doctors says he's much better off inpatient. If something happened at home that required hospitalization again, he'd have to go by ambulance to ER where, in the past, he had to wait nine hours to be seen, and they do not allow visitors in ER.

Has anyone else had this experience of not having one good reason for such a drastic decline without growth of the tumor? I'm heartbroken. I never imagined that once he entered the hospital this time he would never be coming home! What happened?

* * *

Dear friend,

I am truly sorry for what you and your husband are going through. Your message is very tough to read because I can so clearly imagine all the pain experienced throughout this hard saga, probably because my son went through something similar.

The factor you may be missing is that damage from the disease is one thing, but damage from all the treatments that are applied in order to extend life as long as possible can be almost as bad.

Radiation, for instance, can cause a brittling of blood vessels in the vicinity of the tumor which then degrades the functioning of certain parts of the brain. The heavy dosages of steroids can cause irreversible cognitive and physical impairments. Avastin can be rough on the system too, leaving its own degradation of cognition and mobility in its wake. And some of these treatment effects can come on rapidly—basically when the brain gets to the point when it says, "I have had enough!"

In short, you are witnessing the collision of the disease and the treatments for the disease. That's what happened.

It is the most difficult and most unpredictable art for the doctors to know how much of what treatment to provide to a person in order to extend their life to the maximum extent while at the same time keeping an eye on the quality of their life. Sometimes the disease and their own response to the treatments do not give doctors many choices. From what you have written about all the setbacks, I think your husband's doctors had nothing but choices between bad and worse. All they could do was try what they did.

It is good that your husband is in an inpatient hospice, because if it was just yourself caring for him, it would be impossible to give him the care he should have in the late stage of this disease. Still, I am very sorry about this outcome and am sending my strongest wishes that you are able to find some bit of consolation through this and that your husband has the gentlest, most compassionate ascent possible.

Jana

* * *

Another person wrote in, and Jana was there once again....

Dear friend,

I am so very sorry for your heartbreaking, repeat loss to this nasty disease.

You are entirely right that GBM treatment has not advanced meaningfully in the last several decades. Much research has been done, but it has yet to bear the kind of fruit that makes a difference to us in real life.

Probably the looming reason is simply supply and demand. If a person has $1 million to donate to research that looks for a cure for a cancer that kills 150,000 people each year (lung cancer) or one that kills 18,000 each year (brain cancer), which do you donate your money to? How about if you are a pharmaceutical company with some capital for research and development, which disease do you try to tackle? Our rarity makes us the poor sister who gets the worn-out hand-me-downs.

But there is another aspect. In the last decade, scientists have realized something difficult about brain cancer research. It cannot be done in the standard way, which is to inject lab rats with GBM, give them drugs, and see what works. Almost none of the drugs developed using this traditional method have worked for brain cancer. In 2019, we started the year with six highly promising treatments, and by August all but two had failed, and the remaining two had done so poorly they were not expected to go anywhere.

Scientists have realized that the environment of the human brain is unique, what with its blood-brain barrier and this matrix that what works in the lab almost never works in real people. What researchers now realize they have to do is construct brain organoids in the lab, infect those organoids with GBM, and then test the drugs. This is a super expensive process and one so complex that only premier labs can do this work. So, not only is brain cancer rare as cancers go, but it is immensely complex and expensive to research. I could go on, but you get the idea. Brain cancer research is like the last medical frontier. Fortunately, brain cancer research can sometimes take advantage of research done on other cancers (from which we can get some repurposed drugs) but only sometimes.

But another reason is this: human suffering from brain cancer is relatively unknown to the rest of the population. People will go "ooh and ahh" when they hear of a diagnosis because they connect the diagnosis with the worst, but that's as far as they understand the disease. They have not a clue what daily, even hourly horrific devastation it can bring to the patient and their families. Heck, most of the people fighting this most complex and all-encompassing disease here cannot even get a case manager assigned to them by the doctor's office to help them with the myriad of real challenges they experience. And according to doctors I have gone to on my knees with this issue, it all comes down to a lack of funds.

Without understanding this disease and what it does, there is no priority for donations, for research, or support when and as we need it. Sometimes I think we need someone to make a movie of dealing with GBM for a year to two so that people can get educated and thereby be encouraged to help. Otherwise, as long as we remain in the dark, this scourge will continue, and, 30-40 years from now, you may be asking the same question.

Again, I am so sorry for your loss, and I applaud your courage in the face of your pain to see what can be done to spur improvements in treatment so that other wives do not have to experience what you just did.

Jana

* * *

Please help. I am a single mother of two. I just got home from the hospital. I'm doing well getting around; however, mentally with my memory and minor things, I'm struggling. I am in a bad spot financially, and I don't want to lose my home, and I want to give my two girls the best Christmas.

* * *

Hello. My wife has glioblastoma, and she was diagnosed in August of this year. She is 100% bedridden and can't talk or chew, but one of her eyes is open. No facial expressions at all. She will also hold my hand. We talked to many surgeons, and none can operate on her. We have her using Optune, which I do not agree with at all. It was developed for active people with glioblastoma, not those in her state. We started giving her ashwagandha powder in her shakes. Anyone have experience with this holistic treatment? Will it save her life?

* * *

My father was diagnosed with grade IV glioblastoma in July and has since gone through two brain surgeries, one to remove the tumor before radiation treatment and the other shortly after radiation because a part of his tumor recurred to the side of where the radiation treatment actually was. Given the fact that this disease is so unpredictable (as it has shown us with the recurrence right after radiation), does anyone have any experiences to share with recurrence?

To add, where my dad's tumor is, it sits right where his speech and complex thinking are. He has barely any short-term memory, but his long term is still there. He has difficulty communicating about certain things and also gets frustrated because of it. His right side is weak because the tumor is on the left side of his cerebrum.

Feel free to share experiences and advice. He is a man who can't sit still and is upset he can no longer do the things he used to. He has also refused to get any further treatment at this time. There were no current clinical trials he qualified for that were around our area either. I feel absolutely terrible for him as he is not the same person on the outside but still very much is on the inside and can't express himself fully. It breaks my heart.

Thank you.

Holly Richard

* * *

Our life has changed, and emotions are very high. All I hear echoing in my ear is rare, untreatable, and glioblastoma. What is this and what are the next steps? Mom was rushed to the hospital in November and admitted to prep for her biopsy where it was diagnosed. She has high grade, level 4, fast growing brain cancer (Multiform A GBM).

I keep hearing surgery will take away her quality of life, radiation, and chemotherapy will not cure her, but it may slow it down and shrink it a little which will help with her headaches and quality of life.

It's a lot and to me the process seems to be moving slowly as I keep hearing stage-4 echoing in my head. To me that means no routine. Mom is scheduled for another CT scan today.

I'm here to surround myself with people who understand my crazy emotions, may want to share their experiences dealing with this crazy disease and resources to help my family get through this.

* * *

Dear friend,

Researchers may have just, in the last six months, found that one common thread. But before I give you the punchline, I just want you and anyone reading this to have an appreciation of just how immensely hard finding any commonality among GBMs is.

There are, as best as we understand today, four different types of GBM: proneural, neural, classic, and mesenchymal. Each of these subtypes is radically different from the other.

The mesenchymal is identified by a loss of CDKN2A and NF1 genes, an expression of SERPINE, TRADD, RELB and CTGF, plus the presence of these biomarkers: CHI3L1, METY, CD44 and MERTK.

The classical is identified by amplification of chromosome 7 (many have an extra chromosome 7), chromosome 10, EGFR amplification, NES expression, and CDKN2A deletion. Note that CDKN2A loss happens with both mesenchymal and classical, but that's where the similarity stops.

The proneural has IDH-1 point mutations. (I think soon, like maybe 2021, the World Health Organization will re-categorize brain cancers and those with mutations of the IDH-1 will no longer be called GBMs but rather Anaplastic Astrocytoma Grade 4. Just a small percentage of GBMs have a mutated IDH-1, and the outcomes for them are significantly better than those where the IDH-12 gene is unmutated.). Proneurals also have PDGFR alterations, and they have mutations in the TP53, DLL3, DCX, TCF4, SOX, ASCL1, and OLIG2 genes.

Neural subtypes over express for GABRA1, SLC12A5, SYT1, and NEFL.

In short, there is basically no common thread to be found even among the four known subtypes of GBM. Certainly not as these subtypes are currently defined.

But, as I started this message, researchers just recently found what you may be looking for. There was a research study conducted by Hui Li, PhD, of the University of Virginia School of Medicine and the UVA Cancer Center. Li and his colleagues stumbled onto a protein that shows up in 100% of GBMs. It is called Advillin or AVIL for short.

This protein comes from a gene that is part of a family of genes that produce actin regulatory proteins. AVIL binds to actin, and I guess that action sets up the process whereby a GBM ensues in due time.

Yes, the researchers found in their lab that when they silenced the AVIL gene so that it does not produce its protein, all the GBM cells in the lab got wiped out. (Note that wonderful things that happen in the lab do not always translate into the same occurrence in the human brain, but this one could be The One.)

AVIL appears to be a bona fide oncogene, appears to be involved in 100% of GBM cases, and appears to be a terrific therapeutic target. Maybe it is the common thread you were looking for.

Jana

* * *

Hi all,

Today was a difficult day in our tangle with the great brain monster. My wonderful husband is on Avastin (infusion 11) and has really lost a lot of mobility in his left side in the last four weeks. He had an MRI yesterday, and I managed to get a conversation with his NO [neuro-oncologist] today. It was horrific because she insisted on an in-person conversation, but because of COVID, only my husband could go in, and I had to listen by phone. She basically looked at the latest MRI and said that, along with clinical symptom presentation, it means that he has about six months left and that we could do Avastin if we wanted but that she is referring us to palliative care. He can't do any chemo or Dex because he has a skull defect (skin pulling away from incision) from a previous infected bone flap removal, and low WBC counts will promote infections.

I feel terrible for all the usual reasons but especially because my husband was so surprised by this. He told me that he thought that he had longer. Now I feel like I shouldn't have asked the questions that led her to say outright that he only has six months to live. I feel like I've somehow burst his bubble of absence of info that kept him optimistic, and I am just so sad that I feel like I will never climb out of this well of despair. I had to ask these questions because my husband is deteriorating so rapidly that I don't want to wake up one morning and find that he can't move at all, and I haven't prepared for it.

I don't have a question. I just wanted to scream into this safe space for a few minutes before I put my game face on and act cheerful and positive.

* * *

My mother was recently diagnosed and was told surgery is not an option as it is too diffuse. I believe that is the correct way to say it. Too imbedded. Radiation and a chemotherapy pill are options, but they will only possibly improve her quality of life for the little time she has left. Can anyone offer insight as to what this means? She is so weak now, cannot walk as her right side is affected and is incontinent. Wouldn't radiation and chemo make her weaker?

Holly Richard

* * *

Dear friend,

Oh, this is so hard. First of all, I am so sorry this disease has found your mother. Secondly, the whole notion of putting an older, fragile person with a terminal cancer through treatment is simply daunting.

You should know that there are no established standards for GBM treatment in individuals of your mother's age. There are just so many concerns like underlying health issues, fragility due to age, and immune system compromise that have to be considered on a case-by-case basis.

That said, there have been studies that have shown radiation (with the concurrent low dose chemo) is safe for elderly patients. The chemo, which is Temozolomide or Temodar, is given in a low dose and is generally tolerable, but most people who get it are not always your mom's age and do not always have her deficits.

In cases where there is a doubt because of the person's underlying health issues, some doctors will prescribe three weeks of daily radiation instead of six weeks.

Candidly, I would have a couple of conversations or, even better, one conversation at the same time with at least two experts present. One person I would want to have a really candid, Dutch uncle kind of conversation with is the radiation oncologist. I would want to hear about his/her expectations of how your mother is likely to react to radiation and what the reasonably anticipated implications are if your mother has no radiation or has just half of the normal treatment.

The other person I would want to talk with is a palliative care counselor to understand how best to keep your mother comfortable if she gets none, some, or all of the radiation/chemo treatment.

Then, before doing anything, you need to have a conversation with your mom to share with her what you learn from these experts and to understand what her preferences are. If your mom wants to make a full court press, throwing all available medical intervention at her cancer, then no matter what, you should support her.

Similarly, if she just wants to allow the disease to progress naturally, then you support her in that. This disease has robbed her of all sorts of options, but the one she still has is the option to handle this challenge her way, and, as caregivers, we have to be ready to offer our loved ones the dignity of having their wishes supported.

I get that this could be a conversation that is immensely difficult to have. If so, you can pull in a resource like clergy, a trusted friend, or a level-headed family member to help facilitate it. But ultimately, the decision is hers, so it's important to know what she wants to do. My heart goes out to you. This would be very hard for anyone.

Jana

* * *

For those that know about my wife with GBM, we are in the eighth month now, and she is in hospice care. We stopped feeding her two days ago. My heart is broken after 30 years of marriage to the most perfect wife! Thank you for all your support! It's up to Hashem now! God bless all of you going through this horrible experience!!

Holly Richard

* * *

After a very long fight with a GBM, my 32-year-old daughter passed this morning in her sleep. She fought each and every day over the past 20 months to live. I continue to pray for all who have watched their loved ones struggle through each day of this horrific disease and will continue to pray for you and your loved ones.

Chapter 20
Joe's Mom

I met Mary Ann, Joe's mom, shortly after Derek was diagnosed with glioblastoma in the underground world of the brain tumor community website, *Inspire*. This is also the place where I met the mothership of *Inspire*, Jana, who has also shared several writings in this book about her son Aaron's cruel and courageous battle with glioblastoma. Aaron passed away on January 18, 2015. He was 31 years old. I asked Mary Ann if I could include her son Joe's equally cruel and courageous battle with glioblastoma, and she agreed. With all of the attention that mental health is getting today (thank God!), I felt Joe's battle with GBM is one that needed to be written and blasted from the mountaintops for all of the healthcare providers around the world to hear. This is her story.

My son Joe was a typical, albeit exceptionally bright, sophomore who was attending college at a local university in March 2011 when he decided it was his duty to contact all the department chairs to help them realize they were off base in their approach to education. He undertook his activity on a Friday afternoon, so, fortunately, the deans and department chairs were not around. But his behavior didn't go unnoticed, and, although he ended up back at his fraternity house playing video games, the Department of Public Safety (DPS) showed up to remove him in handcuffs for a trip to the psychiatric emergency room. And so his journey began.

Policies on campuses protect students' privacy, so parents cannot be notified when such an incident occurs, but Joe's father had been a prominent faculty member before leaving the university, so he was called and then notified me. Joe's brother was a junior on the same campus, and, although parents could not be called, Joe's brother was contacted, and he rode in the back of the security car and waited in the emergency room. It was late on a Friday and the ER was filling with patients who had destabilized and would be seeking shelter for the weekend. Several hours after I arrived, my son was taken in a wheelchair with two orderlies via a tunnel system and elevators up and down to the inpatient unit, and I was told that I could not stay with him.

Joe looked at me and said, "Mom, *One Flew over the Cuckoo's Nest!*"

He had taken an elective course in high school on the language of film, so I understood his reference and responded, "And two of us landed, baby."

Although, as a nurse practitioner, I knew more than most people about healthcare and hospitals, this was my first encounter with having a family member admitted to an acute psychiatric unit on an emergency basis. I asked friends and colleagues for treatment protocols. Both the Department of Defense (DoD) and VA protocols start with brain imaging, so at the first opportunity I asked his psychiatrist, who was the head of the department, about getting a fasting functional MRI.

He said, "We'll get to that."

They never did. It turns out that insurance companies create a great deal of red tape for a mental health provider to get even a CT scan approved, so no one ever looked at Joe's brain during that episode. Nor was one performed the following year after another incident, which was worse and ended up with Joe being committed by court order to an institution for over a month. During both of his extended treatment periods, Joe spent weeks in isolation and was even restrained because no one could control his behavior.

For the last two years of university, there were no incidents, Joe was not on any medication, and received no further treatment. He made the Dean's List every semester and was inducted into the Economics Honor Society and went on to graduate school.

In the spring of 2015, Joe completed his master's degree in economics and was living the independent life of a graduate assistant, keeping office hours, grading papers, moderating exams, and trying to figure out his dissertation focus. Then in the fall, just after Halloween, he fell off the cliff of mental illness. Again, he was manic, and his behavior became concerning to those around him. Again, word came to me via one of his friends, as his privacy was protected over his well-being. His psychosis persisted despite his withdrawal from classes on medical leave and frequent, sometimes daily, visits with the psychiatrist at the student health center until he flew to the East Coast for the holidays. On Christmas Day, he was again taken with law enforcement's help to an acute psychiatric unit.

As the ambulance drove away, the officer in charge asked, "What is your son like when he isn't sick?"

His brother and I assured him that Joe was the nicest, kindest person you would ever want to meet.

The officer responded, "It is a good thing you had this set up as a psychiatric emergency because, otherwise, we might have hurt your son." He was shaking his head as he left our home.

A week later, after Joe finally agreed to see me since his illness made me either a victim or a villain, I left and drove cross country to a new job in California. As I drove, I wondered if I would ever see my youngest son again.

Joe remained in the hospital for less than two weeks, and, when he was discharged, he flew to his dad's house in the Midwest because insurance was refusing to cover his care. Again, without much treatment, Joe recovered. He was working out daily and enjoying cooking with his dad and playing with his younger half-brother until he began experiencing excruciating headaches the first week of February. I previously reported Joe's episodes of headaches to his father, stepmother, and the nurse coordinating his visits to an outpatient psychiatrist. No one seemed concerned; the headaches came and went, and arrangements were made for Joe to fly to California to spend a month with me.

He arrived on a Wednesday evening, smiling, backpack slung over his shoulder, headphones around his neck, and eager to see a desert landscape as we drove home. March was always a time we enjoyed because of NCAA basketball, and we watched a game. Joe started to get settled into this environment. We sat in the hot tub in the yard under the star-filled sky and talked about the national park, where he could work out and just hang out. He asked for some Tylenol for a headache. He said maybe he had eaten something bad the day before and went off to sleep. The next day he was fine but again felt sick to his stomach but made no big deal about it. Friday, he called me at work, saying he had lost his balance in the hot tub but was okay, and then a couple of hours later he called and said, "Mom, come home now; I am really sick."

In the remote desert town near the military base where I worked, there weren't a lot of services, no urgent care, and the ambulance I called said it would take them longer to get to us than it would for me to get to the small hospital in the next town.

By the time I pulled up to the emergency entrance, Joe couldn't walk. I called for help, but again, on a Friday afternoon, the ER was very busy. Someone pointed me to a wheelchair, and I managed to get his 6'3" lanky frame into the chair, signed him in, and then rushed to move my car before he was called to triage. As the nurse asked the routine questions, he was losing the ability to speak and leaned to one side in the chair. He was quickly taken into the emergency department where there were no beds, but we were allowed an area in the hallway where nausea overcame him, and he began projectile vomiting, which got him into a cubicle. I watched as he began gesturing and speaking in what is known as "word salad" of both garbled words and unintelligible sounds. As he became more distressed, I looked at him and saw his pupils were almost fully dilated. I asked him, "Can you see me?" to which he shook his head no.

I was sure my son was having a stroke and was going to die right then. I conveyed my concerns to the nurses but was met with the statement, "These psychiatric patients can do that sort of thing." Their assumption was he was toxic on lithium, but his level came back so low that the doctor said, "Is he even taking any lithium?"

Attempts to get him into the CT scan were difficult, but, with sedation, the imaging was done, and the doctor who came on the evening shift said: "You have got to see this; there is something in your kid's head."

Within minutes I was following an ambulance with lights flashing, siren blaring, to a hospital where Joe would finally get an MRI. Finally, the source of Joe's behavioral problems was seen: a tumor in his left thalamus. Surgery revealed it to be a glioblastoma (GBM). They gave him two years to live. I shared a case study nearly identical to Joe's history to the neuro intensivist in the ICU who commented, "We see this all the time." The nurse navigator at UCLA shared with me that her father had been written off as dementia before his tumor was found.

It took a few months, but finally his medical record was corrected to show he did not have bipolar disorder, and he had been misdiagnosed.

At the cancer treatment center, he met with the social worker who asked me tearfully, "What did they do to him in the psychiatric hospital? Joe said being treated for cancer is better than being a psychiatric patient."

I told her, "You don't want to know."

Joe was vindicated. He said, "I told them I wasn't bipolar."

I will always wonder *what if*. What if brain imaging had been done when he had his first episode of mania when Joe was 19? If they did and the pediatric neurosurgeon operated on Joe, would it have killed him, or would the tumor have blown up earlier if they did any sort of treatment? Or would he have had treatment and been given a few more years? We will never know. But now, when I hear that someone with mental illness is killed on the streets, I wonder, "Did anyone ever do brain imaging to see if that person had a tumor?"

Joe passed away on January 12, 2018. He was 27 years old. Joe didn't get to finish his PhD, but his brain did go to UCLA for research. It is the best we could do. There are two scholarships and one research fund that bear his name. Something good has to come out of something bad. But did my son have to suffer the indignities in the mental healthcare system, the stigma he experienced on campus when all the girls moved to the other end of the bar when he sat down, and, most of all, I wonder why everyone with his type of brain cancer has to die.

Chapter 21
An Ode to Brain Cancer,
Aaron's Mom

This poem by my friend Jana speaks deeply to my heart.

An Ode to Brain Cancer
In memory of my son, Aaron

For the startling news that makes something break inside and
the mind go blank,
For the shock that makes the ground under one's feet shake,
For the sleepless nights and cold sweats,
For the fear that makes one come face to face with oneself,
I cry.

For the hours spent in waiting rooms and days with stomachs
empty and knotted, waiting to hear results,
For the desperation mingled with hope that chases second and
maybe even third or fourth opinions,
For the consuming distraction of precious time and energies,
For all the ruined hopes and expectations, sadness and pain,
I cry.

For the little ones watching, confused and anxious,

Holly Richard

*For the spouses, significant others, parents, grandparents, and
other loves ones who cry in the middle of the night when no one
can see,
For the friends who don't know what to say so they say nothing,
For the relationships that get gnarled or lost along the way,
I cry.*

*For degrees that can't be completed and jobs that can't be kept,
For damaged futures and finances, insurance hassles, and
insensitive bureaucrats,
For the social workers and therapists that couldn't help,
For scam artists and charlatans that come to prey,
I cry.*

*For the engagements, weddings, births, and birthdays never
celebrated,
For cancelled vacations or vacations that could not be planned,
For the homes never bought and those that had to be mortgaged,
For the shattered dreams of life left undone,
I cry.
For the hurtful words said by the frightened or well-meaning,
For the indignities of hair that falls out, surgical scars, the bruises
from infusions and blood tests,
For the unwanted looks of pity on peoples' faces,
For the restrictive diets and food favorites that shouldn't or
cannot be eaten anymore,
I cry.
For nerves that go numb,
For the arms and legs that are too weak to work properly,
For the nausea and fatigue, misguided taste buds, impaired
vision,
For the confusion and erasures of memories,
For drug-spawned moodiness and words not meant,*

For the eyes clouded and pained by pounding headaches,
For the desperation that grows into depression,
I cry.

For long-term survivors who are living proof there is a reason to
hope,
For the loving caregivers who emerge from all backgrounds, and
learn with a robust determination to take care no matter what,
For kind friends who can be trusted to call, to bring food, flowers
and encouragement even when others may have faded away,
For those amazing people who just seem to know how to bring
a comforting perspective and help us let go of what we cannot
control but fight for what we can,
For the unbreakable relationships forged or strengthened in the
heat of this disease,
I celebrate.
For the people who gave up years of fun and freedom to study so
that they could help those with brain cancer,
For those MRI and rehab technicians, infusion nurses, and
surgical staff who do their work with utmost care and humanity,
For the social workers who offer their shoulders and provide
helpful assistance,
For the prayer warriors who plead relentlessly,
For hospice staff who lower the stairs of Heaven a bit when those
steps are just too tall for us,
For the grief-stricken who swallow their pain of loss and lend
support to those fresh to the brain cancer journey,
I celebrate.
For extraordinary courage and resilience shown by those in the
brain cancer community over and over and over again,
For those who get up each day bravely focused only on that one
day,
For the kisses and "I love yous" that do so much to comfort the

spirit,
For the numerous complaints that are justified to be voiced but
are left unsaid for the sake of peace,
For those whose character and principles are not eroded by this
disease,
For those who refuse to see themselves as powerless and waiting
for brain cancer to work its worst,
For those who live in the darkness of this disease but still shine a
bright light in this world,
I celebrate.
For those pure souls, sparks of God, who are tethered to the
physical challenges of brain cancer's fury, but refuse to be
identified solely by their diagnosis,
For their courage toward themselves and for their compassion
toward others despite their own weighty concerns,
For Faith that is tempest-tossed and tested but not broken,
For Grace that allows one to stand with strength or that brings
angels to lean on,
For Hope that permits one to see beyond the reaches of this
disease,
For Love that endures above and beyond all brain cancer and
never, ever goes away,
I celebrate.

—*Jana, mother of Aaron*

Chapter 22
Love and Grief

Derek's heavenly 30th birthday is today, March 26, 2021, the second birthday without him here. April 10th will be the second year since I had that ambulance ride with Derek, taking him to hospice, followed by April 17th, which will be two years since he passed. April 22nd was the day we had his funeral two years ago. I had no idea how to put a title to this poem, so I left it alone.

How does a mother say happy birthday to her child
Who was laid to rest before her eyes?
How do I even say happy
When I had to say goodbye?

Nothing makes sense, you should be here;
The table is still set for you;
Your chair is there and you are not.
My heart still broken in two.

Holly Richard

In the quiet hours of early morn,
I can hear you whisper,
"Mom, please do not cry,
Remember me and live for me
As I have lived 10 times."

Yes, you have, my traveling son,
Taking me with you to those faraway places,
With your FaceTime calls from around the world,
Precious memories, exhilarating faces of life's races.

And so I say happy birthday my son.
How proud I am to be
The chosen one, to be your mother
And the forever bond between you and me....

All my love,
Mom
© 2021 Holly Richard

* * *

Two years ago today, April 10, I was in the back of the ambulance with Derek on the way to hospice. Seeing his unresponsive body, so thin and fragile, started revving up in my mind. The panic rose over and over again. I remember thinking, *How could this be; how could he be dying?* Why was I in the back of this ambulance with my son who 118 days earlier was making music and getting ready to watch the ball drop on New Year's Eve and heading to college a couple weeks later? What the hell was happening? I heard the beeping as the ambulance backed into the entryway to the hospice unit. That sound, beep, beep, beep, beep—would it ever stop?

* * *

On April 17, 2021, we visited the cemetery, Nic, me and Dave. In memory of Derek, I posted the following note to my Facebook page and to Derek's.

To all of our friends and family,

It is hard to believe that two years ago today our precious Derek passed away. We continue to miss him so much, yet we know we must go on and live life to the fullest as Derek did every day. We know that is what Derek wants for us, and we know in our hearts he will always be with us.

Our family continues to honor and remember Derek, and, if you would like to, here are some ways you can do so:

- We memorialized his Facebook page, so feel free to visit and post a message any time.
- We have a memorial website you can visit at https://www.

forevermissed.com/ and type in Derek's last name, *Lemieux*, in search. You can post pictures you may have with Derek, post a tribute, or simply view the site at any time.

- May is Brain Cancer Awareness month and is when people can wear the color gray in memory of all of the people who have lost their lives and show support to those who are living with brain cancer.

- Save the date for Angels Among Us' 5K run and Walk of Hope on October 2, 2021, at Duke. We hope it will be in person vs. virtual. We will be putting together our second D-Rex Defenders team soon and will send out more information and a link on how you can join and/or donate. It will be a day of celebration and hope for patients, friends, and families whose lives have been affected by brain cancer. These critical funds will support cutting-edge research being done at the Preston Robert Tisch Brain Tumor Center at Duke Hospital in Durham, North Carolina, where Derek spent months receiving treatment.

We thank you again for the amazing support we continue to receive from so many people.

Much love and appreciation,

Derek's family

* * *

April 23, 2021

I have given all I can give to this book, I think, and now it is time to write its ending. I do not know where my grief journey will take me. I was going in the opposite direction and then was thrown onto this path. There, I have met countless of parents who have lost their child in so many gut-wrenching ways. I am so sorry. Their losses are all way too soon, and we all end up in the same place, the same space, walking on the grief journey's path without the physical presence of our beautiful children. That out-of-order death electrocutes, debilitates, and oftentimes leaves us raging, in denial, or dry heaving on the floor. When the pain isn't so loud, I crave to listen to Derek's heart and presence.

It has been a long, hard two years and counting. I have witnessed the unimaginable and have come to realize that all of what I have written and all that Derek experienced, along with my family and friends, really did happen. I know I will continue to experience grief at different times and in a variety of ways for the rest of my life until I am reunited with Derek again. We love our children immensely; therefore, our grief is just as immense. For me, grief and love must line up parallel to one another like a train track. Left track: immense love; right track: immense grief. The train cannot go forward, cannot leave the station, unless both tracks are aligned. I find I cannot move forward in life, let me repeat, move *forward*, not move *on*, until I accept the two tracks are together as one, inseparable, just like my love for Derek and his love for me. I feel a bit of movement, I am starting to inch forward....

Chapter 23

Warriors and Arsenals

Here are some ideas and suggestions, and I am sure I missed some that I may not be aware of. These warriors and arsenals are from my family's experiences and what we learned along the way. Regardless of what type of brain tumor, it is in one's brain, and therefore every scenario needs to be thought about and constantly vetted and reviewed.

1. Warriors come in all shapes and sizes. If you have people close to you who can give you a respite, pull shifts if needed, bring you food and other stuff needed to survive the day or night ahead of you, line those people up! In the hospitals, we found the social workers and chaplains supportive and helpful. The medical team and everyone from housekeeping to nurses to docs at both WakeMed and at the Preston Robert Tisch Brain Tumor Center at Duke at were all warriors!

2. Remember, you, the patient, and your loved ones are the mightiest warriors. Make yourself a part of the treatment team as you will be getting your minor degree in becoming a hospitalist! If things are going too fast and are confusing

and overwhelming, call a meeting with your medical team and ask what additional warriors and arsenals you may need.

3. Arsenals: Reach out to the American Brain Tumor Association (www.abta.com) and the National Brain Tumor Society (https://braintumor.org/brain-tumor-information/theexperience/). They work every day to ensure we have a forum for discussion and the dissemination of information, and they serve as the focal point for raising funds so badly needed for research.

4. In the USA and the UK, there are Facebook groups called Bereaved by a Brain Tumour and Brain Tumour Charity Group. There are online brain tumor community groups via Inspire (www.inspire.com). Inspire is partnered with the American Brain Tumor Association and is the site where you can find the mighty duo of Jana, the mothership, who shares boatloads of information and support, and Mary Ann, the other half of this dynamic duo, who shared her story in a chapter of this book. She also lost her precious son Joe to this cancer beast, and she is constantly working behind the scenes to help. She is helping to develop a DNA biomarker to a treatment drug-matching database. There are many other incredible, loving, and supportive people on these sites along with moderators who can help you navigate through your journey while trying to connect you to others who have been or are standing in your shoes. There is also the Mayo Clinic website (www.mayoclinic.org). These websites provide resources and opportunities to share with others who have been impacted by brain cancer. They let you know what they have done, what works, what doesn't, who were/are their medical experts to treat brain tumors and in which states. You can find options for treatments, clinical trials, health insurance

coverage, and places that can help financially. You can talk to people who can share their life experiences of living with a brain tumor as their loved ones care for and support them.

5. Here is a letter straight from Jana, the mothership of *Inspire*. She describes the first four things she feels need to be included if you or your loved one has just been diagnosed with GBM.

Dear friend,

I assume that your husband has recently been diagnosed. Getting a diagnosis like this is something not a single one of us ever expected. After my son was diagnosed, I remember waking up in the middle of the night, night after night, with a jolt like someone had thrown a vat of ice water over me. It hurt to breathe, to pray, to eat, to do much of anything. I couldn't even believe it because he was otherwise so healthy. Nothing made sense.

So, let's see if we can begin to make this make some sense for you. There are four first things (and about 1,000 things after that, but let's start with the first four).

> If your husband has just been diagnosed, you may be in a state of semi-shock, so there's little point in getting into too much detail about GBMs and their treatment until you can breathe again. Tell me when you're ready, and I will inundate you (with probably more than you ever wanted to know about GBMs.)

> Bring all the love you can. Make a point of telling your husband every day how much you love him, appreciate him, and admire him, etc. Don't let the opportunity go by without embarrassing yourself by over-loving him.

> Recognize (as I am sure your gut does) that your

husband has a platinum level cancer; he needs to be treated by platinum level doctors at a platinum level clinic. Maybe the doctor he currently has is someone he trusts with his life. Good. Keep that doctor but build his medical team to include a platinum level doctor. (We can get into the details of how to do that.)

➢ Know that to hear he has a GBM is not the whole diagnosis. Each GBM has its own unique molecular structure and traits. That means each GBM will have its own responsiveness to treatment, its own treatment options, its own prognosis. When you want, we can dig into the details to help you better understand the exact enemy you are up against.

Like other incredible people here have said on Inspire, you are not alone. You can lean on us, and we will help you—at least from an earthly perspective. It will be God who will provide the strength, the wisdom, the perseverance, the patience, and the peace in the midst of the storm that you will need to get through this.

I am sorry this disease has struck your husband and send my strongest hopes that he has the best outcome possible.

Jana

6. Brain cancer clinics: These were put together by Jana in hopes they will be able to give you options when brain cancer strikes and second opinions.

    1. Mayo Clinic, Rochester, MN

2. Johns Hopkins, Baltimore, MD

3. University of California at San Francisco Medical Center, San Francisco, CA

4. Cleveland Clinic, Cleveland, OH

5. New York Presbyterian–Columbia and Cornell, NY

6. Massachusetts General Hospital, Boston, MA

7. Barnes Jewish Hospital, St. Louis, MO

8. Northwestern Memorial Hospital, Chicago, IL

9. University of Michigan Hospitals, Ann Arbor, MI

10. University of California Medical Center, Los Angeles, CA

11. Rush University Medical Center, Chicago, IL

12. NYU Langone Hospital, NY

13. Hospitals of the University of Pennsylvania, Philadelphia, PA

14. Stanford Health Care/Stanford Hospital, Stanford, CA

15. St. Joseph's Hospital and Medical Center, Phoenix, AZ

16. Cedars-Sinai, Los Angeles, CA

17. Mount Sinai Hospital, NY

18. University Hospitals Cleveland Medical Center,

Cleveland, OH

19. MD Anderson Medical Center, Houston, TX

20. Duke University, Durham, NC

21. Jefferson Health—Thomas Jefferson Hospitals Philadelphia, PA

22. Brigham & Women's Hospital, Boston, MA

23. UT Southwestern Medical Center, Dallas, TX

24. Ohio State Hospital Wexner Medical Center, Columbus, OH

25. Mayo Clinic, Phoenix, AZ

26. Houston Methodist Hospital, Houston, TX

27. Beaumont Hospital, Royal Oak, MI

28. Keck Hospital of USC, Los Angeles, CA

29. Indiana University Health Medical Center, Indianapolis, IN

30. University of California, Davis Medical Center, Sacramento, CA

7. For people who have been denied clinical trials because they have not been approved by FDA but could give hope for a cure or some sort of quality of life, attempt to utilize a Right to Try law, and contact the Right to Try Foundation (www.righttotryfoundation.com).

8. The Phase 2 trial for Berubicin for recurrent GBMs is now open. You can see the official trial descriptor at this link, which includes the name/phone/email data for the points of contact: https://www.clinicaltrials.gov/ct2/show/NCT04762069.

9. This site may be able to find options for new clinical trials to treat GBM: https://www.cityofhope.org/breakthroughs/checkpoint-inhibitors-plus-car-t-shows-promise-for-glioblastoma-?utm_campaign=MKT_NTR_Supporter_Breakthroughs_CheckpointGlioblastoma_20210513&utm_medium=email.

10. After his sister-in-law passed away from GBM, Dr. Al Musella began the Musella Foundation. He has provided important resources for many years to the GBM community. He arguably created the first website devoted to brain cancer back in the early to mid 1990s and still maintains a nonprofit foundation that does many things to help brain cancer patients and their families. Here's his website: https://virtualtrials.org/musella.cfm.

Grief Resources:

Below are some resources that I hope may help your aching heart:

1. Compassionate Friends, the world's largest self-help bereavement organization, offers support to grieving family members following the death of a child. Part of their work is to help others be supportive, and they offer assistance to anyone outside the family who wants to help. This non-religious organization is in almost every state, and many states have several chapters.

2. Helping Parents Heal is a Facebook page and a nonprofit organization whose mission is to help grieving parents support one another throughout the healing process. As Jana, the mothership of *Inspire*, expressed in her letter to another mother in chapter 19, one of the ways to survive this maddening grief is to be of service to others who walk the same path. Helping Parents Heal gives us a way to connect and become "Shining Light Parents" to those who share the journey. There is also a FB page for widows and widowers of GBM.

3. Grief Counseling: I swear by my counselor, but counseling may not be for you, and that is okay! Each of us goes through this devastation in our own way and at our own time. For me, after two years and counting, my grief counselor, Mitzi Quint, LCSW, PLLC, continues to be my angel, my life preserver, my candle in the darkness. Her website is https://www.mitziquint.com.

4. Many hospice organizations offer grief counseling at no cost.

5. Bereaved by a Brain Tumor: This Facebook group offers a mutually supportive space for those who have lost loved ones to a brain tumor and those whose dear ones are nearing the end of their journey as a result of this disease. This private groups gives us a chance to share our stories and all aspects of our journey.

6. Grief support groups can be helpful for some people, and they were for me, especially in the first few months after Derek passed. I attended one for a while called Growing thru Grief, which was held at a church in Durham. I loved how they split us into smaller groups with a trained facilitator in each group. I learned so much from the people in these groups about the stages of grief and the different kinds of losses.

7. One of the most therapeutic things I found on my grief journey was participating in writing classes with a group of people, sharing all sorts of emotions based on various prompts, and readings from the facilitator for me.

Acknowledgments

Nic, my beautiful daughter, fought every day for her brother, never giving up, taking such good care of Derek, and was a fierce protector and advocate. She did all of that while also trying to support me the entire time. I love you to the moon and back; you are my everything. Thank you, Nic.

My husband Dave somehow was always there to help with Derek and his care and still be there to support me and Nic. He worked long days and took shifts at the hospital after work and on the many weekends in the mornings so I could get a bit of respite. Dave cried with me and held me when I thought I would die and supported me when grief became my full-time job. He is the love of my life, the one who listens to me scream and sob, and he continues to have more patience than a saint. You are my rock, my best friend, and my everything. Thank you, DJ.

Thank you to all the WakeMed and Duke Hospital warriors who fought alongside Derek throughout this battle with brain cancer for all the love and care you gave to Derek and our family. You are all heroes.

Thank you to Transitions LifeCare for the love and care you gave to Derek and our family.

To our family, friends, and co-workers who sent prayers and food, who came to visit, thank you.

Thank you, Alice, for loving Derek and welcoming him into your family's home to celebrate the holidays while he was stationed in Italy. I know he fell in love with you, and he was your first *amore*. I smile at the photos and memories you both shared and will cherish them and you always.

Thank you to Derek's friends and Army buddies for visiting him in the hospitals and in hospice and for saluting and honoring him at his funeral.

Thank you, Jana and Mary Ann, for sharing your wounds openly and painfully in this book. Your strength and advocacy work help so many people. You are amazing. Both of you and our sons, Derek, Aaron, and Joe, have helped me somehow find the courage to write this book.

Thank you to my cousin Lori, who is always there for me and Nic, and to cousin Shez and her precious daughters, Amelia Rose and London, who carry on the Derek Dab, thank you.

Our Chaplain Luis and wife Linda, thank you for being there day in and day out, bringing Derek's favorite candy, and praying with us every day.

To Mary Freeman, my trusted friend who stayed with Derek at the hospital when we needed coverage on occasion and brought Derek Cook Out burgers, chicken fingers, and peach shakes, thank you.

Thank you to our dear friends, Bob and Sam, Connie and Laurie, Chris and Lauren, Jeff and Laurie, and all our Mardi Gras friends who helped us in so many ways during this time and continue to do so.

To all the grieving moms I met along this journey with whom I have shared my loss and grief and who have shared theirs with me, I am so grateful for each of you. Thank you for the thoughtful texts every year when "that day" comes. As we all say, this is not a club you ever want to be in, yet here we are together, and I am so grateful for each of you.

My angel and grief counselor Mitzi, you saved my life and fought with me and for me and for Derek so I could begin to move forward; you helped me get through this book as I relived the horror. Thank you for helping to make sure Derek and this momma's beast won the battle with the Tumorator tumors as I continue my war with them, exposing them for the world to know and see. I pray this book moves people to take action in the fight to find a cure for this horrific cancer, as Jana calls it, "the platinum level cancer."

To my amazing editor, Diana Henderson, who is a gift, thank you for getting through this book with me, crying with me, and for your immense talent that went into this book. My publisher Drew Becker, what a gift you are too. To be able to read, digest, and gently walk me through *One Hundred and Twenty-Six Days* to get it ready to print over the past several months was an enormous task that I could not imagine, and you did it with such kindness and patience. Thank you.

There are so many people, and it is impossible to name them all, but you know who you are, and our family is forever grateful for your love and support. And finally, to my Derek, thank you for your courage and your love for us to keep fighting to the very end. Thank you for the immense love and memories you have to me. Being your mom has been the greatest gift of all. Until we reunite, I will keep you in my heart, my precious, beautiful soldier son.

Author Bio

I quit high school in my junior year at age seventeen and moved twelve-hundred miles from home with my boyfriend. We rented a home, I passed my GED, and off to work I went. A few years later, we married and had our two children, Nicole and Derek, who were and continue to be my diamonds in the rough and my everything. I thank their father for giving these beautiful children to me to love and cherish.

I began my career in the disability field in the early 1990s, working with individuals with intellectual and developmental disabilities (IDD). This experience was the catalyst for me enrolling in college while working and raising my two children and earning my bachelor's degree. My husband and I divorced after a 27-year sprint of trying to make it all work. You can't say we didn't try.

Over the past 20 years, I have served in executive leadership roles for several nonprofits. During this time, I found my soulmate and best friend, Dave. He also dedicates his lifelong work to advocating on behalf of people and families. We married in 2012 and I was blessed to inherit my bonus child, Dave's son, Dylan.

Holly Richard

Having the honor to be a part of some amazing organizations has given me the inside view of the ironclad lifeline between parents and their children. These brave-hearted parents along with the courageous parents I have met in my grief journey have given me the courage to write this book.

Contact e-mail: hollyj1962@yahoo.com

Website: https://www.drexdefenders.com

CPSIA information can be obtained
at www.ICGtesting.com
Printed in the USA
BVHW070412161221
624023BV00012B/1222